Child and Family Policies

Child and Family Policies

STRUGGLES, STRATEGIES AND OPTIONS

edited by
Jane Pulkingham and Gordon Ternowetsky

We are grateful to the Employability and Social Partnerships Program
(formerly National Welfare Grants) Human Resources
Development Canada (Project #4572-10-90-001) for financial
and program support it provided for this publication.

The views expressed in this publication do not necessarily represent
those of the Employability and Social Partnerships Program.

Fernwood Publishing • Halifax

Editing: Donna Davis
Design and production: Beverley Rach
Printed and bound in Canada by: Hignell Printing Limited

A publication of:
Fernwood Publishing
Box 9409, Station A
Halifax, Nova Scotia
B3K 5S3

Fernwood Publishing Company Limited gratefully acknowledges the financial support of the Ministry of Canadian Heritage and the Nova Scotia Department of Education and Culture.

Canadian Cataloguing in Publication Data

Main entry under title:

Child and Family Policies

> Includes bibliographical reference
> ISBN 1-895686-60-1

1. Family Policy -- Canada. 2. Child welfare -- Government policy -- Canada. 3. Canada -- Social policy. I. Pulkingham, Jane.
II. Ternowetsky, Gordon.

HV700.C3R47 1996   362.82'8'0971   C95-950336-6

Table of Contents

Part 3: Child and Family Poverty:
Evaluating Income Support Programs and Policy Options

Part 4: Advocacy and the Politics of Influence

Part 5: A Postscript: The New Canada Child Tax Benefit

Acknowledgements

As we write these acknowledgements there is a flurry of activity around issues such as child poverty. These include designs by the federal and provincial governments to adopt a new national child benefit plan, and recommendations by groups such as Campaign 2000 that the federal government adopt a life cycle, social investment fund for children. It is also timely as issues discussed in this book, such as First Nations control of child welfare and the provision of adequate funding for First Nations self-government, are highlighted in the recent Royal Commission on Aboriginal People. In addition, provincial reforms currently taking place in social assistance and social services will have a profound effect on children and families. This restructuring is addressed in this book, and we are hopeful that the discussion we present will contribute to a more informed, caring and less punitive approach to social service reform.

We are grateful to a number of people for assisting us in the completion of this book. First of all, thanks to the contributors for their participation and patience as we placed the completion of this book behind that of *Remaking Canadian Social Policy: Social Security in the Late 1990s* (Fernwood Publishing 1996), another edited volume inspired by papers presented at the Seventh Conference on Canadian Social Welfare Policy held in June 1995.

We are grateful to National Welfare Grants and its successor, the Employability Partnership Program of Human Resources Development Canada, for supporting both the Seventh Conference on Canadian Social Welfare Policy and this book *Child and Family Policies: Struggles, Strategies and Options*. In particular we want to thank Sandra Chatterton, Evariste Theriault and David Thornton formerly of National Welfare Grants. While NWG is gone, we are hopeful that, in the future, we will be able to work with these individuals under the auspices of another federal body devoted to promoting community-based research and developments in Canadian social policy.

A number of other key people were involved in different stages of the planning of the Seventh Conference on Canadian Social Welfare Policy that gave rise to this book. This conference was held in Vancouver from June 25th to 28th, 1995. In addition to ourselves, the organizing committee consisted of Michael Goldberg, Social Planning and Research Council of British Columbia (SPARC of BC); Andrew Armitage, Social Work at the University of Victoria; Roop Seebaran and Frank Tester, Social Work at the University of British Columbia; Stuart Alcock, British Columbia Association of Social Workers; and Dan Smith, United Native Nations. The planning for this conference was greatly facilitated by the administrative and organizational work of Lisa Griffith and Loralee Delbrouck.

Two people helped us with the preparation of this manuscript: Heidi Tait of the Child Welfare Research Centre at the University of Northern British Columbia and Vicki McKendrick, the Social Work secretary at UNBC. Throughout the course of editing this book, Heidi and Vicki assisted us with many details such as typing letters, sending faxes to the contributors and inputting the text. We would also like to thank the folks at Fernwood Publishing—Errol Sharpe, Donna Davis, Debbie Mathers, Beverley Rach, Brenda Conroy and Lindsay Sharpe.

We want especially to thank our families for their forbearance and continued support for yet another year of longer work hours and time away from home. Edward and Liam, Carroll, Alex and Joe inspire us in many different ways, all of which find expression in the way we have been able to undertake and complete this book. Finally, our thanks to one another for spurring each other on and making the process an enjoyable one.

Jane and Gordon, December 1996

About the Contributors

Jane Pulkingham is a professor of sociology in the Department of Sociology and Anthropology and past director of the Social Policy Issues Post-Baccalaureate Diploma Programme in the Faculty of Arts at Simon Fraser University. Her teaching and research interests are in the area of feminist political economy of the welfare state, gender and social policy, employment and income security policy and family law (economics of divorce and child custody determination). She has recently edited with Gordon Ternowetsky *Remaking Canadian Social Policy: Social Security in the Late 1990s* (Halifax: Fernwood Publishing).

Gordon Ternowetsky is a professor of social work at the University of Northern British Columbia. His research and teaching interests are in the area of unemployment, poverty and social policy and social work. He is the founding editor of *Australian Canadian Studies: An Interdisciplinary Review* and a former editor of *The Canadian Review of Social Policy.* He is the coordinator of the Child Welfare Research Centre at the University of Northern British Columbia. He has also edited, with Graham Riches, *Unemployment and Welfare: Social Policy and the Work of Social Work.* Toronto: Garamond.

Maureen Baker is a professor of social policy in the School of Social Work at McGill University. In addition to teaching in several institutions in Canada and Australia, she was a social policy advisor to Parliament from 1984 to 1990, and is now involved with cross-national research on family policies.

Karen Callahan recently graduated with a bachelor of laws degree from the University of British Columbia and is currently completing her articles. Following a teaching position in Japan, she completed her master's degree in English at U.B.C. in 1993. Her thesis analyzed the images of women in children's literature.

Marilyn Callahan teaches child welfare, community development and social policy in the School of Social Work at the University of Victoria. Her doctoral thesis *Stereotypes of Women in Child Welfare* examined images of women through an analysis of historical documents and media coverage. Her latest research explores the experiences of mothers in child protection investigations. The article in this volume is the first joint publication for mother and daughter, an academic partnership they hope to maintain.

Evelyn (Lyn) Ferguson is an associate professor in the Faculty of Social Work at the University of Manitoba where she teaches feminist social policy analysis and social work practice. She has been doing research in the area of child daycare policy for ten years and is particularly interested in parental preferences and involvement.

Diane Gray-Withers has a master's degree in public administration from the University of Manitoba/University of Winnipeg, specializing in social policy reform. She is currently working for the Manitoba government on the social policy renewal process. She has been active in a number of different community development initiatives and is now focused on creating a Legal Aid and Safety Centre for women in abusive relationships.

David Hay is the senior research associate at the Social Planning and Research Council of British Columbia (SPARC of BC). His doctoral thesis examined the relationship between income and health and was completed at the University of Toronto in the Department of Community Health. His current research interests include social welfare, theory and practice. He recently published with Marcia Rioux *Well-Being: A Conceptual Framework*.

Steve Kerstetter first started writing about social policy as a reporter in the Ottawa bureau of the Canadian Press wire service. He joined the National Council of Welfare in 1988 and has been director of the council since 1995.

Julia Elissa Krane received her doctorate from the University of Toronto in 1994. An assistant professor at McGill University School of Social Work, she teaches and engages in research on violence against women and children from a feminist critical perspective. Her current projects include the completion of a book on child protection practices in cases of child sexual abuse, and two research investigations into the provision of culturally sensitive practices in shelters for battered women.

Clarence Lochhead is the director of the Centre for International Statistics at the Canadian Council on Social Development. His publications include *The Canadian Fact Book on Poverty* and *A Statistical Profile of Urban Poverty*.

Susan McGrath is a doctoral candidate in the Faculty of Social Work at the University of Toronto. She has taught social policy and community practice at Ryerson Polytechnic and McMaster Universities. She has been active in several social advocacy organizations including the Social Planning Council of Metropolitan Toronto, and has been a member of the steering committee of the Child Poverty Action Group since 1989.

Brad McKenzie is an associate professor in the Faculty of Social Work at the University of Manitoba, where he teaches in the areas of social policy, evaluation and child and family services. He has completed a number of studies on community-based services and child welfare issues in First Nations communities. He is currently co-editor of the *Canadian Social Work Review*.

Susan Prentice is a member of the Department of Sociology at the University of Manitoba. From 1993 to 1996, she held the prairie-region Margaret Laurence Chair in Women's Studies. She has researched childcare issues, and been active in childcare advocacy since the early 1980s.

Glen Schmidt is an assistant professor in the Department of Social Work at the University of Northern British Columbia. Before joining UNBC he worked for the University of Manitoba Social Work Access Programme located at Thompson in northern Manitoba. His social work practice is largely in child welfare and mental health where he has worked extensively with First Nations people.

Part 1:
Introduction

The Changing Context of Child and Family Policies

JANE PULKINGHAM AND GORDON TERNOWETSKY

Introduction

The studies reported in *Child and Family Policies: Struggles, Strategies and Options* consider feminist and First Nations critiques of child welfare, policy options for child and family poverty, and studies of the politics of influence in child and family policies. The argument presented below is that economic and political factors set the context for understanding the making and unmaking of social policies in Canada. The purpose of this chapter is to provide a framework for understanding the way these factors influence the problems considered in each of the studies included in this volume.

The first objective of this introductory chapter is to review briefly the economic circumstances that set the stage for the making of social policy during the 1980s and 1990s. This review considers different layers of economic change that precipitated the growing demand for state intervention in a period when governments are winding down public provisions for collective well-being. In doing so, the discussion draws on the articles in this book and provides a framework where the issues presented in these papers are linked to material influences that have shaped recent policy making in Canada.

There are, of course, several jurisdictions of policy making in Canada. Federal, provincial and territorial governments enact social policies and, in the area of families and children, many have programs in place. There is also the evolving First Nations jurisdictional control of child welfare services, an issue that is addressed in several of the contributions to this volume (see Gray-Withers 1997, McKenzie 1997, and Schmidt 1997). For the most part, the discussion in this introduction is limited to the federal arena because, in terms of the funding arrangements of welfare policies in this country, the role of the federal government is crucial for understanding policy developments in Canada.

A second purpose of this introduction is to consider the influence that neoliberalism, the dominant ideology of our times, has and will continue to have on Canadian social policies. As Baker (1997:159) demonstrates, "political ideology remains the decisive factor in explaining the development of social and economic programs." Selected economic and social policies that took hold in the 1980s and 1990s are reviewed. What seems clear is that "paralleling" the growth in need during these years is an emergent view that social policies are "no longer affordable, just at the time they are most needed" (McDaniel 1993:74). The discussion illustrates that the Mulroney-style neoconservatism of

14

the mid-1980s to early 1990s, and the later day neoliberalism of the Chrétien Liberals, are essentially the same in terms of prescriptions for growth, prosperity, the proper role of social policy and a sentimental reconstruction of the "traditional nuclear heterosexual family" (Coontz 1992; McDaniel 1993; McGrath 1997). This discussion suggests that the deteriorating economic and labour market security witnessed since the early 1980s ushered in an era of federal social security reform and cutbacks that have further "shaken" the security of the people in this country (Lochhead and Shalla 1996:19).

The value of such a discussion is that it pinpoints influences that will affect the making and remaking of social policies in Canada in the foreseeable future. Whether related to broad issues such as employment and unemployment or specific policies in the area of children and families, ideological forces sway the way society chooses to deal with social and economic issues of the day.

The third and final section of this chapter uses the framework provided in Mishra's (1990) study of welfare states in capitalist economies to show that, in the key areas of employment and unemployment, universality and selectivity and safety net provisions, the retrenchments initiated by Mulroney's federal Conservatives were later consolidated by the Chrétien Liberals. In terms of safety net provisions, however, the new Canada Health and Social Transfer (CHST) has fundamentally altered the Canadian welfare state (CWS). The shift to a block funded CHST from the conditional funding of the Canada Assistance Plan (CAP) means more power but less money for the provinces and territories, fewer national standards and disappearing mechanisms for enforcing standards.

These outcomes are in keeping with Canada's shrinking federal or centrist welfare state. The context of social policy in the late 1990s is one in which the economic vulnerability of families and children is being met by increasingly decentralized, minimalist and residual state welfare within a globalized economy dominated by transnational corporations. This retreat compounds the economic insecurity brought on by labour market restructuring and the collapsing structure of opportunity. Yet the impact of this retreat is uneven.

Some would argue, for example, that it is children who are ultimately most affected by the accelerating insecurities confronting families (Lochhead and Shalla 1996:17). To a certain extent this perspective informs policy recommendations and the strategies adopted by advocacy groups such as the Child and Poverty Action Group (discussed by McGrath 1997), and coalitions such as Campaign 2000 (discussed by Hay 1997 and Baker 1997 respectively). Certainly when family security is undermined, so are the well-being, opportunities, life chances and futures of children. However, to single out children in this way plays into existing distinctions between the "deserving" and "undeserving" poor. It obscures the extent to which the process of labour market and welfare state restructuring is gender-, race- and class-based (Brodie 1995; Fraser and Gordon 1994; McDaniel 1993) and brings specific pressures to bear on "improperly constituted families" (Callahan and Callahan 1997:53) in an attempt to reconstruct a traditional family form (McGrath 1997:170).

Struggling for Security:
The Economic Context of Insecurity

In a recent Forum on Family Security (Ross et al. 1993:1, 2) the "central issue of our times" is reported to be the "insecurity felt by families, their children and their children's families." In looking at this struggle, this section surveys recent changes in employment, unemployment, underemployment, inequality and poverty which suggest that the structure of opportunity for an increasing number of Canadians is in decline. This changing opportunity structure constitutes an important layer of influence that undermines the security of Canadians. Equally important are factors, such as changing family forms and structures, that mediate the way market based insecurities are dealt with and felt by families and children.

The circumstance precipitating the insecurity of Canadians over the decades of the 1980s and 1990s are well documented (Pulkingham and Ternowetsky 1996a; Department of Finance 1994a, 1994b; Ross et al. 1993, 1996; Bellemare 1993; Ternowetsky and Thorn 1991). The view presented here is that the restructuring of labour markets sets the context within which the struggle for security occurs and can be best understood. This is illustrated when the following changes in unemployment are considered.

In the post-war period and prior to 1982, the official annual rate of unemployment exceeded 8 percent twice, during the recessions in 1977 and 1978. Since 1982, in contrast, the average annual rate of unemployment has risen steadily and has fallen below 8 percent only twice, in 1988 and 1989. Unemployment rates that were once rare are now commonplace as joblessness remains at historically high levels in both good and bad economic times. Indeed the 8 percent level that was once uncommon is now the norm. As noted by the federal government, the "core rate" or "benchmark of full employment" is "at least 8 percent" unemployment (Department of Finance 1994a:20).

Today this means unemployment that exceeds 1.2 million people is natural, unavoidable and acceptable. Companies in pursuit of profits and a competitive edge, as well as governments attempting to control deficits through spending cutbacks, are shedding staff, creating unemployment and offsetting potential employment growth. While the current Canadian government treats the resulting levels of high unemployment as unavoidable, through policies such as the new Employment Insurance (EI) legislation (Bill C-12) it is also screening people out of jobless benefits by curtailing access through entitlement changes.

It needs to be noted that official unemployment figures underestimate the real level of joblessness in Canada (Social Planning Council of Metropolitan Toronto 1985; Ternowetsky and Riches 1990). Left out of these official counts are people who have dropped out of the workforce, discouraged workers who believe jobs are not available and have stopped looking for work, and First Nations people living on reserves. When these are included the real level of "acceptable" joblessness in Canada is 15 percent, representing more than 2.2 million persons in the labour force.

Underemployment, in part reflected in the rate of involuntary part-time employment, also constitutes a form of joblessness not captured in official rates of unemployment. Approximately 28 percent of part-timers work part-time involuntarily (Krahn and Lowe 1993:94). In addition, a much larger proportion of part-timers (almost one-half) are involuntarily working fewer hours than they would like (Duffy and Pupo 1992:69).

Combined with the insecurity brought on by unemployment and underemployment is growing long term unemployment and the restructuring of work (Human Resources Development Canada [HRDC] 1994a). The latter is modifying the face of Canadian labour and the level of economic security that traditionally accompanies paid employment. The restructuring of work is reflected in the shift to the service sector from jobs in the goods producing sector, the growth of part-time, non-standard, contingent labour, and the increasing share of women in the workforce. It is what these trends have in common—lower wages, fewer benefits and less job and income certainty (Department of Finance 1994a)—that is problematic in terms of the security and well-being of Canadians.

These converging trends in unemployment and employment signal the end to a level of economic security the majority of workers and their families once took for granted. The restructuring of work means that market successes and economic growth no longer translate into enough jobs of sufficient quality to ensure decent living standards. The evidence pointing to these outcomes is increasingly plentiful. At a general level examples of this restructuring include the stagnation of average family earnings and the decline in living standards. For example, the share of earnings as well as after tax income levels for families with children fell for the bottom three quintiles or 60 percent of families in the 1980s and early 1990s (Maxwell 1993; Ross, Scott and Kelly 1996). This precipitated both a widening of income inequality and a decline in middle incomes. It is the drop in the share of income of the bottom second and third quintiles that best depicts this declining middle. Between 1984 and 1993, the total income of this middle 40 percent of families with children went down by 4.5 percent. Their average, after tax incomes dropped further by 8.1 percent. On the other hand the earnings of the top two quintiles went up, reflecting the growing polarization that is characterized by a lot of poor paying jobs, and fewer good jobs with good pay (Lochhead and Shalla 1996:17, 18).

In response to falling family incomes, women in dual partner families have entered the paid workforce in increasing numbers. Today, approximately two-thirds of wives are in the paid workforce, a rate that increased substantially in the last twenty years (Lindsay 1992:27). Their labour force participation has not only helped families maintain accustomed living standards, but their participation in the paid labour force has more than halved the percentage of two parent families that, without this extra income, would be in poverty (National Council of Welfare [NCW] 1996:83).

The latest poverty figures still show, however, that some 349,000 two parent families with children are poor. What is instructive from these data is that the major source of income for 57 percent of these families comes from earnings and EI (NCW 1996:8). It is clear that their poverty cannot be attributed to low work commitments, an increasingly common refrain in today's era of policy making. On the contrary, what these findings indicate is that both the unavailability of secure and stable paid employment (as witnessed in the persistent high levels of unemployment), and low pay (which characterizes the new job market), are the major factors that keep families in poverty.

Lochhead's (1997) study on policy options for low wage workers affirms this conclusion. He argues that the "new economy" of high unemployment and the expansion of low wage work ensures the persistence of the working poor. He also cautions that low wage work should not be viewed by policy makers as a stepping stone to better jobs and wages. On the contrary, his study reveals that, over a three year period, more than 60 percent of low wage workers, the majority of whom are women, "remain at the same level, moved down or out of the labour force" (1997:141). What the expansion of both unemployment and low wage work guarantees is a "growing permanent class of working poor" (1997:134).

When individual and family security is undermined, so is the economic security of children. Child poverty, which for a short period in the late 1980s was declining, is once again rising. Recent figures show some 1.4 million children in poverty, up from the 934,000 children that were poor in 1989, the year the House of Commons passed the all party resolution to eliminate poverty among Canadian children by the year 2000 (NCW 1996:11; Campaign 2000 1994a). Child poverty is the result of family poverty that is pushed up as employment and good paying jobs become harder to find. These same factors also force families onto public assistance, where the inadequate levels of income support reinforce their economic marginality and ensure the persistence of poverty among families dependent on public assistance (NCW 1996).

We also know that children from lone parent families have a much greater chance of being raised in poverty. In 1994, 57.3 percent of lone parent families were poor, compared to 11.3 percent of couples with children. When desegregated by the gender of family heads, 70 percent of families headed by women are poor. This rate goes up to 81 percent for lone parent mothers who were never married (NCW 1996; Ross, Scott and Kelly 1996:3).

Several points can be made concerning the circumstances of security and insecurity faced by parents and children in different family structures (Lindsay 1992). First, although the rate of growth has slowed, the number of lone parent families is rising. Between 1981 and 1995, lone parent families increased from

11 percent to 14 percent of all families. The rate of increase was more marked for never-married lone parents: in 1981, one in ten lone parents were single never-married. By 1995, one in four (25 percent) fell into this group. In contrast, the once dominant family form—married couples with children—is now less common. From 55 percent of all families in 1981, it dropped to 45 percent in 1995 (Statistics Canada 1996a). Second, most lone parents (82 percent) are women, a major factor leading to the feminization of poverty. Third, compared with two parent families, the economic circumstances of lone parent families are far worse and since 1980 have deteriorated more rapidly (Crompton 1996; Lindsay 1992). The level of dependency on government transfers is one indicator of this. Among two parent families in 1994 transfers account for 8 percent of their total income, in contrast to the 31 percent for lone parent families. For families that are poor, between 1982 and 1994 government transfers comprised 33 percent and 61 percent of two and lone parent family incomes respectively (Crompton 1996:44). Among lone parent families government assistance is a vital source of income for the poor as well as the non-poor. Fourth, economic insecurity is not simply about income distribution, it is also about the distribution of time. There is a need for more adequately remunerated working time for the unemployed and family time for parents. Families face considerable time constraints in juggling childcare and work. This is especially acute for single parents who face the dilemma of opting to not work at all (ensured poverty) or working very long hours to be able to both afford childcare costs and justify (financially) participating in paid work. The availability of adequate, affordable and accessible childcare and extended parental leave arrangements together are key to ensuring greater economic security: both are necessary to provide greater support for participation in paid work as well as choice in how domestic caring responsibilities are arranged.

The above discussion indicates that economic insecurity has become commonplace during the 1980s and 1990s (Ross et al. 1993, 1996) While labour market restructuring and its attendant outcomes are primary sources of this insecurity, family structure and form influence the way in which economic insecurities are dealt with and experienced. These in turn are shaped by social policies which may alleviate, exacerbate or create social and economic insecurity.

To a large degree, family structure is a "problem" only in the context of anachronistic policies. These arise out of a set of contradictory prescriptions rooted in the attempt to privatize (individualize) responsibilities, through the "family" and/or the "market." Notably, these contradictions are most apparent where systems of child welfare, social assistance, family law and childcare intersect. One of the most enduring anachronisms is the fashioning of entitlements, programs and support predicated on the nuclear heterosexual norm and the male breadwinner family wage model. "This model operates on the assumption that women's financial needs should be met ... through men's participation in the 'public sphere' of paid employment and their direct relationship to the state" (Pulkingham 1995:2). Relatively few families consist of a sole breadwinning husband, stay-at-home wife and children. Nevertheless, provisions across a spectrum of policy fields, including social assistance, child welfare, childcare and child support, assume that mothers' employment is peripheral; they are available to undertake (unlimited) unpaid caring work; and they are and should be supported by male partners.

These principles are revealed in social assistance regulations and practices, for example the "spouse in the house" rule, which limit women's independent access to benefits if a man is living under the same roof. Another example is requiring separated and divorced mothers to pursue child support orders and support enforcement in order to be eligible for social assistance. This practice is widespread among the provinces. Here the state is extending its powers to impose by force mothers' financial dependence on ex-spouses through the compulsory enforcement of child support awards. More broadly, child support is a key mechanism by which the federal government claims to address children's economic rights and reduce child/family poverty. In the 1996 budget (Department of Supply and Services 1996), the federal government announced a new child support package consisting of four key areas: three of these pertain to child support (tax treatment, guidelines and strengthening of enforcement procedures) pursuant to divorce; the remaining area is enhancing the Working Income Supplement (WIS) of the federal Child Tax Benefit (CTB) (discussed below in the section "Universal Social Programs"). The significance of this package is twofold. First, at a time when the federal government is busily offloading financial and provisioning responsibilities for social programs to the provinces, this is one arena in which it is enlarging its sphere of activity (redirecting financial resources to this area, administration and legislation). Second, however, the federal government is not increasing direct financial supports for children and families. Rather, it is entrenching its ability to enforce private responsibilities, whether these are familial obligations to provide financial support (child support) and/or individual obligations to engage in paid work (WIS).

In the child welfare arena, the "motherhood mandate" (Prentice and Ferguson 1997) is reflected in forced unpaid motherwork to protect children from abuse (Krane 1997, discussed in more detail below). This flows from the presumption of a mother's innate capacity and duty to care and protect (Callahan and Callahan 1997; Jiwani 1996), even where it is clear that she is unable to do so. This issue is explored in Callahan and Callahan's (1997) analysis of the press coverage of a public inquiry into the circumstances surrounding the death of Matthew Vaudreuil at the hands of his mother. The motherhood imperative is also reflected in childcare services. Not only is childcare largely used to replace motherwork in the home, "[e]vidence that childcare services substitute for mother-care is encoded in legislation which stipulates that childcare subsidies are only available if (both) parents work or study" more than a certain number of hours a week (Prentice and Ferguson 1997:200).

Simultaneously, these assumptions coexist with competing ones. For example, social assistance reform, intent upon ending the "cycle of welfare dependence" and disincentives to work, is reformulating work requirements so that a larger proportion of lone parents (the vast majority of whom are mothers) are designated as "employable" (Evans 1996; Scott 1996a; Phipps 1993). In tandem with the rise in the proportion of lone mothers reliant on social assistance, mothers increasingly are being treated "the same" as other categories of recipients. Motherhood no longer confers "deserving" status, difference-based entitlement or protection from the market (Pulkingham 1996; Vosko 1996; Scott 1996a; Fraser and Gordon 1994). As in other arenas (e.g., unemployment insurance reform) the requirement to work (the "employable" designation) is being fortified, regardless of domestic caring responsibilities (Pulkingham 1996) and the availability of services and supports to help accomplish these competing demands.

In the child welfare arena, the motherhood mandate also is differentially applied in class and race specific ways. On the one hand, there is the case of Verna Vaudreuil (see Callahan and Callahan's chapter) which points to the imposition of the motherhood imperative regardless of the capacity to mother/ parent. On the other hand, there are many families, a disproportionate number of whom are poor and/or First Nations, for whom the norms of good mothering/ parenting are consistently negated, reflected in high rates of child welfare apprehensions (Gray-Withers 1997; McKenzie 1997; Schmidt 1997). As Callahan and Callahan (1997:41) argue, "[w]omen, particularly poor single women, are seen to be doing a bad job of looking after children. Welfare bashing of single parent women has become common . . . and sensational child welfare stories feed the myths of women on welfare."

Women simultaneously resist and accommodate the "norms of 'good mothering'" (Prentice and Ferguson 1997:201) and the competing pressures and inconsistent policies flowing from the attempt to shore up private responsibilities. Fundamentally, however, the "private solutions" mothers create reflect the overwhelming pressure to be responsible. The whole institution of motherhood and mothers' expectations of themselves" places pressure upon them to conform to unrealistic expectations (Prentice and Ferguson 1997:200; Krane 1997; Callahan and Callahan 1997).

A major challenge for policy is to redress labour market insecurity and accommodate different family structures with their diverse issues, needs and resources. Another task is to respond to emerging pressures for culturally appropriate policies that address the unique circumstances of First Nations people. At one level policies geared toward creating good paying jobs, expanding the opportunity for paid employment and providing universal benefits and services are needed to address the general issue of widespread economic insecurity. At a second level there are pressures for supplementary, selective programs and supports for targeted groups, for example lone parents, who have fewer resources for dealing with economic insecurities. There is, in addition, a third level policy response for First Nations where, alongside programs and services for addressing general economic insecurities and the needs of targeted groups, culturally appropriate policies designed and controlled by First Nations are in order.

In terms of the first level, the evidence reviewed in this chapter points to a definite need for universal policies to respond to the growing levels of economic vulnerability experienced by increasing numbers of people. However, in the face of these pressures, it is difficult to mount universal programs in today's era of policy making. McGrath's (1997:175) chapter reminds us that in this "neoliberal" era of "debt and deficit reduction" we are being pressured by governments and the corporate sector to expect less from our social programs. In this climate the principle of universality is being abandoned by social policy groups on the left and the right as "too expensive." As noted in McGrath's chapter, there is now considerable political support for developing a national child benefit to combat child poverty. In this period of restraint it is likely that this benefit will be income tested and targeted to low income families with children even though economic insecurity is increasingly widespread. According to McGrath (1997:179) the Child Poverty Action Group (CPAG) is one of the few remaining policy groups that has retained a universal element in its proposed child benefit. This universal component, however, is in the form of a "tax credit" rather than a direct income transfer, a position that "reflects the pressure to remain relevant" to the demands of the current neoliberal policy environment.

An example of the second level of targeted support is reported in Kerstetter's (1997) chapter "Fighting Child Poverty with Parental Work Income Supplements." Tackling the issue of the much criticized work disincentive of welfare, that recently has gained so much credence across the country, he examines a model that provides supplements of $3000 for lone parents and $4000 for two parent families. While the proposed supplement would remove work disincentives for lone parents in most jurisdictions and single earner couples in four provinces, and augment work incentives for two earner couples, this strategy is not without problems. Kerstetter (1997:155) concludes that income supplements are "no substitute" for "more and better jobs," reduced unemployment and "affordable and accessible childcare." The other caveat is that the model is based on minimum wages that, except for two earner couples, are so low that they keep people in poverty. As noted by Lochhead (1997:143) these minimum wage levels reinforce a "permanent working class" and thereby intensify economic insecurity. What this suggests is that the issue of work disincentives lies in the labour market, with its low minimum wages, rather than the benefit levels of welfare (Clark 1995:2). In other words, targeted polices are of questionable benefit outside of a policy framework providing universal benefits, services and jobs with adequate pay.

At the time of writing there is considerable discussion about a new, national child benefit plan to reduce the number of children in poverty. Although national, this is an example of a second level targeted policy option. While discussions are still preliminary, several key components seem to have emerged. On the one hand, the new national child benefit would involve federal and provincial cooperation in the financing and administration of the new plan. On the other hand, at this stage, this new benefit is based on enhancing the existing federal CTB, although it appears this will be accomplished, in part, by better targeting benefits to the poorest families with children (Greenspon 1996b:A6). What this means for other families in economic need, but not deemed to be in poverty, remains unclear.

A further component hinges upon the provinces' willingness to divert social assistance funds currently paid to families with children into this national child benefit. Whether the provinces will pursue this is not certain, although there is growing momentum to permit different provinces to design alternatives that best suit their current needs and provincial priorities (*Globe and Mail* 1996b:A20). One preferred option that has emerged includes making welfare less attractive than work. Such initiatives usually involve providing extra income or incentives to the working poor such as the BC Family Bonus (discussed below) that is paid only to working families with children and excludes families with children that are unemployed or on social assistance. Other incentives contain extending benefits normally paid to welfare families to families that are in the workforce. These include benefits such as medical and dental coverage which are usually eliminated once families no longer receive social assistance.

While the extension of benefits is important, denying benefits to families because they have no member in the workforce is inappropriate. This is the case as it ties benefits designed to help children to a parental work test. It is also inappropriate as it reinforces the distinction between the "deserving" or working poor and the "undeserving" poor who are not in the workforce. Another point, as discussed above, is that it is time to reconsider the issue of work disincentives or the "welfare trap" as lying in the labour market, with its low minimum wages, rather than an outcome of welfare levels and benefits that exceed wages.

Another approach suggested by the Campaign 2000 (1996a) coalition is to develop a life cycle, or social investment fund for children that could be funded by current government expenditures on child benefits, a progressive tax on total income and corporate contributions. This incorporates many elements of a first level universal approach to eliminating child poverty. The principal features of this fund include a comprehensive child benefit system, a financial package for provinces to support childcare and early development initiatives and an education endowment plan that sets aside $20,000 for the post secondary education of children from working class families. It is the comprehensive child benefits system that aims to reduce Canada's current child poverty rate. The benefit has three components: the enhanced basic child benefit that "would reduce economic hardship for all poor families and bolster the living standards of modest income families"; the Family Care Supplement geared to increasing the subsistence level incomes of parents with children on social assistance; and the Advanced Maintenance Payment System for Child Support, a public system of protection that, like Employment Insurance which protects the loss of wages, would protect the loss of living standards for women and children "who lose the contributions of a separated earner" (Campaign 2000 1996a:4). According to Campaign 2000 estimates, the availability of these funds could lower current child poverty rates by 60 percent and move Canada in the direction of achieving the House of Commons resolution of eliminating child poverty by the year 2000.

A third layer of policies is suggested in the case of First Nations and their struggle for self-government and jurisdictional control over child welfare. As noted in the chapters by Schmidt (1997), McKenzie (1997) and Gray-Withers (1997), among First Nations there is a history of high unemployment, economic dependency, poverty and cultural genocide brought on by white colonization and the Indian Act. These have impoverished and disempowered First Nations communities and their people and have led to a wide range of social and economic problems. Services and programs that are culturally sensitive, adequately funded and controlled by First Nations are a logical next step. As shown in the Royal Commission on Aboriginal Peoples (Parker 1996:B1), centralized, government run programs to date have not successfully dealt with the economic insecurities that have fed the social and personal problems confronting many First Nations communities.

However, a key issue in this process of assuming jurisdictional control over child welfare and other services is the role played by First Nations women. Gray-Withers (1997) points out that First Nations women have been sidelined in this process. Their judgments are quelled both by white male governments that control First Nations and by native organizations that are dominated by men. This tension, addressed in this book, reflects a cross-cultural burden faced by most women in their dealings with the state apparatus set up to protect children. As noted by Krane (1997:59), there is a general silencing of women's voices in "matters" that are rife with consequences for women."

The next sections consider some of the ways the federal government has responded to the struggle for economic security in the 1980s and 1990s. This is addressed in two stages. The evolving ideological context of social policy making in Canada during these years is first reviewed. In the last section, a selection of polices are evaluated using Mishra's (1990) framework for comparing tendencies of social policy retrenchment.

The Social Policy Context of Insecurity

The provision of security "forms the traditional heart" of Canada's welfare state (HRDC 1994a:25). Today this emphasis is particularly apt, given that economic insecurity is widespread and increasingly common. However in the face of these growing economic uncertainties, we have witnessed a winding down and retreat in the provision and access to state welfare in this country. A number of descriptors have been used to depict this withdrawal. Phrases like restructuring, remaking, reweaving, retrenching and dismantling point to both an "erosion" and what others label as a "demolition" of Canada's welfare state (Brodie 1995; McBride and Shields 1993:66, 67; Mishra 1990; Mullaly 1993; Pulkingham and Ternowetsky 1996a; Ecumenical Coalition for Economic Justice [ECEJ] 1993). While there is some debate concerning the extent to which Canada's welfare state has been dismantled (eroded or demolished), there is general agreement as to why this took place in a period of growing demand.

As in other western economies, the factors leading to the restructuring of welfare provisions in Canada are both material and ideological (Mishra 1990). The recession of the early 1980s, followed the oil shock of the 1970s, resulted in high unemployment and inflation and a growing demand for state assistance. These had the effect of discrediting conventional Keynesian solutions for managing the economy. On one front "confidence in the state's ability to manage a mixed economy" collapsed (Mishra 1984:190). This collapse, in turn, opened the way for theories of the right which, in addition to their rejection of Keynesianism, championed policies to limit the scope of the state and reassert market forces. As pointed out by Johnson, McBride and Smith (1994:4), a variety of labels including "the new right," "neoconservatism" and "neoliberalism" are used to describe the approach to governance that has dominated economic and political thought in Canada and other western economies since the early 1980s. Throughout this chapter we largely use the term "neoliberalism."

The main ideological thrust of neoliberalism is the primacy of the market for distributing goods and services and regulating human activity. It is a philosophy that aims to foster circumstances that promote private sector profits and economic growth. The guiding assumption is that a healthy market will benefit everyone. In line with this, the presumption is that profits will be reinvested and wealth and jobs will be created, which in turn will spur further economic growth, investment and job creation. Once again, according to neoliberalism, the problem with the welfare state is that it imposes collectivism, undermines individualism and prevents the market from working efficiently. For example, the burden of taxation required to fund the welfare state creates "market disincentives" (see Offe 1981). Money that would normally be invested in productive capacity and enterprise is channeled into unproductive, welfare state activities. A second set of disincentives is argued to stem from the protection provided through state benefits such as unemployment insurance. The neoliberal objection is that the guarantees offered through these entitlements keep people from working as hard or as productively as they would had they not had access to this protection. In other words, these benefits "insulate" workers, preventing markets from functioning efficiently.

These prescriptions were given political expression in Canada with the election of the Mulroney Conservative Party in the early 1980s. During their tenure, the Conservatives set in motion economic and social policies that reinforced the primacy of the private market. Many of these ideas and policies were later adopted and consolidated by the Chrétien Liberals in the 1990s. This convergence is demonstrated in economic and social policies that have focused on controlling debts and deficits, restraining spending, curbing the influence and scope of government, privatizing public companies, and the remaking of social policies that, it is argued, push up deficits, "produce labour market disincentives and, in today's global market, impair Canada's international competitiveness" (Pulkingham and Ternowetsky 1996a:6).

The social policy changes stemming from these neoliberal priorities have reshaped and redefined the role of the Canadian welfare state. Since its inception the Canadian welfare state has been fluid and changing (Hess 1992). As it evolved, however, its early residual role gave way to one in which it became an integrated, "first line of defense" against market contingencies (Guest 1980:2). In the place of its early, targeted, stigmatizing, means tested benefits, the historical evolution of Canada's welfare state is characterized as a "flight from selectivity" to a growing reliance on universal programs (Banting 1985:9). However, the changes initiated and witnessed in the 1980s and now in the 1990s represent a "reformulation" of many of the values and principles that buttressed the expansion of Canada's welfare state (Courchene 1986). The role of the welfare state is once again becoming residual, with benefits that are less generous, discretionary and targeted. This represents a clear reversal of the welfare state as it has developed in Canada during this century.

In a number of realms, the counterpart of a residualist and non-interventionist state is the obligatory yet invisible unpaid labour of women. As McDaniel (1993:167) argues, one consequence of the rightward direction of social policy is the "feminization of social problems." Instead of pointing to the structural, political and economic bases of a range of problems, the changing structure of families (those that do not conform to the nuclear heterosexual norm) is blamed. Importantly, culpability is centred on women in families.

Women's family and caring responsibilities are closely and inextricably tied to their opportunities for security (McDaniel 1993:164). At a time when two incomes are necessary to maintain average family incomes (Statistics Canada 1996b) and, for an increasing number, maintain an income above the poverty line (as discussed above), reduced government funding for social services is placing an even bigger burden on women. As the state retreats (both ideologically and in its direct financing/provisioning role), women are obliged to undertake more unpaid caring work with respect to partners, children, the elderly, infirm, sick and disabled. Although this work is largely unpaid and therefore remains essentially invisible, perhaps even more imperceptible is the dynamics of this process in the child welfare arena. Here the implications are evidenced at the individual and familial levels. In addition, however, they intersect in a way that women's inadequacies as wives and mothers become a defining feature of the problem (Krane 1997; Callahan and Callahan 1997; McGrath 1997).

One of the paradoxes of neoliberal non-interventionism is the continuation of intrusive forms of social regulation, albeit in a more covert or disguised form. As Krane (1997) demonstrates, in the child welfare arena the public mandate to protect children (operating on the principle of "least intrusion") is misleading in three ways. First, contrary to discourses that present child welfare as a public mandate, in many instances (e.g., cases of child sexual abuse) protection is actually performed by women in the private sphere of the family. As such it constitutes forced, unpaid motherwork. Second, because mothers are not written into the protection mandate explicitly, state practices which depend on mothers to protect are deceptive. State intervention in the guise of "relief for the family" typically entails little respite for mothers who are given minimal material and other supports in taking on this role for the state. Third, regulatory practices of the state are brought to bear on these mothers: the corollary of the obligatory yet invisible protection role of mothers in the home is increased scrutiny and regulation of their activities.

Thus, accompanying the neoliberal welfare state drift, a shift in policy focus to poor children "at risk" is creating new forms of social regulation (McGrath 1997:181). Despite the efforts of child poverty advocacy groups to construct all poor children as "deserving" (regardless of how their caretakers became poor), practices and policies associated with the neoliberal agenda further entrench the prevailing tendency to reframe child poverty as child neglect. Once again, this issue is gendered. For example, "bad mothers" are seen to produce "poor children" (McGrath 1997:181), a particular (improperly constituted) family structure—lone parent mothers—is targeted and its effects are disproportionately felt by poor and First Nations women and children.

The next section of this chapter considers the impact of these neoliberal priorities on the changing character of Canadian social programs during the 1980s and 1990s. How far down the path of neoliberal reconstruction have we gone? How far has the security of Canadians been undermined by a resurgence of residualism in social policy? These questions are addressed by evaluating policy changes in the areas of employment and unemployment, universality and selectivity, and the maintenance of safety net, anti-poverty measures that focus on minimum standards (Mishra 1990:71).

Neoliberalism and Retrenchment: Employment, Universal Programs and the Social Safety Net

In Mishra's (1990:26) analytic framework comparing social policy regimes and developments, the commitment to full employment and the provision of universal services constitutes the "first line of defense" for maintaining national, minimum standards. The second line is safety net provisions for protecting the living standards of the poor and most vulnerable. Regarding the impact of neoconservatism on social policy in Canada during the 1980s, Mishra (1990: 79) suggests that "in the absence of external or internal shock . . . social developments are likely to remain centrist and evolutionary." He recognizes that the dismantling of unemployment policies, universality and safety net provisions have "weakened" the welfare state. In his view, however, these have been piecemeal and the welfare state, after the neoconservative assault of the 1980s, still remains intact.

The analysis presented below suggests that the retrenchments that have taken place since the 1990s have fundamentally altered Canada's welfare state. In the key areas of unemployment policy, universality and safety net provisions the policy momentum initiated by Mulroney has been consolidated by the Chrétien Liberal government. There has been a "flight" from universality to selectivity, declining support for collective provisions, a move towards a decentralized welfare state and a fundamental erosion of safety net protections for the most vulnerable.

Employment and Unemployment

Full employment is a pillar of the post-Second World War welfare state in most western capitalist societies. Although full employment was never pursued in Canada, there was a policy of high (or near full) employment. During the 1980s and 1990s, even this was abandoned and replaced by anti-inflationary employment policies which redefined full employment. In the 1980s full employment translated into an unemployment level of 6.5 percent (Minister of Supply and Services 1985). In the 1990s, the equivalent unemployment rate is 8 percent (Department of Finance 1994a:20). In today's economy, this means that "full employment" is predicated on the existence of 1.2 million unemployed.

The policy response to unemployment in the 1990s reflects the prevalence of a new neoliberal social policy ideology. Accompanying an increasing preoccupation with the setting of market creating conditions, "active" labour market and employment policies and a retreat from the principle of full, or near full, employment, unemployment insurance and welfare reform reinforce the neoliberal fixation with reducing public expenditures, program costs and government deficits and debt. More importantly, these reforms buttress the centrality of the wage–labour obligation and point to the emergence of a gender neutral worker–citizen model (Pulkingham 1996; Scott 1996a; Brodie 1995; Fraser and Gordon 1994).

In the case of unemployment insurance, reform 1990s-style rests on a rejection of the notion that an intensification of non-standard employment should be met with extended coverage and expanded protection. This stands in sharp contrast to the view prevailing in the early 1970s when UI last underwent significant amendment. At that time changes led to increased coverage and entitlement. Under the Mulroney government, a new phase of UI reform was introduced in 1989-90 (through Bill C-21). Although the trend toward reduced generosity began in the mid- to late-1970s (Green and Riddell 1993:S108; Forget et al. 1986), unlike previous reforms, this phase is aggressively pursuing the goal of producing "savings" (containing rising public expenditures and reducing the federal deficit) and "active" rather than "passive" income support.

Privatization of UI is one of the most significant changes introduced with Bill C-21 in the early 1990s. Here the government converted UI financing from a tripartite (employee, employer, government) arrangement, to one financed by employees and employers only. This represents a clear shift from public, collective responsibility to individual responsibility. Privatization of UI is one of the main reasons why Mullaly (1993) suggests that Mishra (1990) underestimates the impact of neoliberal retrenchments on the welfare state. Subsequently, primarily under the Chrétien Liberal government, a range of restrictive changes were implemented, including benefit rate reductions, the imposition of more strict claimant reporting and entrance requirements, penalizing leavers ("voluntary" or through "misconduct") through longer periods of disqualification and reductions in the duration of claims (entitlement rules) (Employment and Immigration Canada 1994). These changes, introduced piecemeal over a number of years, culminated in the implementation of a new employment insurance (EI) system (Bill C-12, July 1996) which replaced the Unemployment Insurance Act and the National Training Act.

The new EI system represents an intensification of efforts already begun in this phase. In particular, there are two key issues—entitlement and coverage—that need to be considered. Importantly, the new EI system will accelerate further the decline in entitlement while it expands coverage. Although UI began as a limited and restricted program, since its inception coverage expanded gradually and now stands at 93 percent (HRDC 1996a: A (2):6). EI will increase this to 97 percent of the labour force, through the inclusion of all part-time workers. But increased coverage and entitlement are distinct issues. Increased coverage is meaningless unless the corollary, entitlement, is also enhanced. While EI will increase coverage, it also imposes more restrictive qualifying rules and eligibility requirements and therefore curtails entitlements. This will accelerate the precipitous decline in the ratio of beneficiaries to unemployed persons begun in 1990. This ratio has already dropped from 87 percent in 1990 (Canadian Labour Congress 1995:2) to 46 percent in January 1996 (Hargrove 1996:A17).

Despite recognition of the increasing precariousness of stable, full-time employment (HRDC 1994b), UI reform, culminating in the new EI system, is a central component of the government's strategy to facilitate market creating conditions pursued through labour market deregulation, reduced wage demands, increased economic insecurity and the discipline of labour (Stanford 1996:137-38, 144).

Universal Social Programs

The principle of universality, reflected in a range of services such as primary and secondary education, health care, public pensions and (formerly) taxable cash benefits for families with children (family allowance), "constitutes perhaps the core element of the post-war welfare state" (Mishra 1990:23). In the "post-crisis" era, however, it is much maligned and beleaguered.

The neoliberal critique of universal programs is that they are an inefficient use of resources in two ways. First, because benefits go to rich and poor alike, they are not adequately targeted to those most in need of assistance (the "poor"). Second, at a time when governments are wrestling to pay down deficits and debts, universal programs are unaffordable. Instead, it is argued that scarce public resources should be selective, targeted through income and means tested benefits, so that only those who truly are the most "needy" receive assistance rather than "wasting" money on those who do not.

The process of undermining universality began with the Conservatives under Mulroney. Over the course of two successive terms in office, the Progressive Conservatives made four attempts to break with the principle of universality. Although the first attempt (1984) was unsuccessful, at least in the immediate term, the effect of subsequent forays was more than symbolic (Mishra 1990; Department of Finance 1984). In the second try (1985), the government proposed the partial de-indexation of Family Allowance (FA) and old age security (OAS), and was successful in accomplishing this with the former. Thus began the era of "social policy by stealth" (Battle and Torjman 1996) where payments increase only by the amount that inflation exceeds 3 percent. This results in a gradual but certain deterioration in the value of benefits.

In 1989, the government proceeded with its third and more serious attack— imposition of a clawback (and partial indexation of the income threshold above which the clawback is applied) on the family allowances of higher income families. A similar clawback also was imposed on OAS for higher income individuals (Hess 1992). Through the benefit clawback, the government undermined directly the principle of universality by introducing an income-contingent component. In addition, the partial indexation both of the income threshold above which the clawback is applied and increases in the benefit ensured that the proportion of families/individuals eligible for full benefits and the value of these benefits would decline steadily over time.

Despite these developments, some would argue that in the 1980s the Progressive Conservatives retreated politically from enacting major changes to universal social programs. Attempts to alter them are variously described as a "fizzle" and a "half-hearted attempt to break with the centrist consensus in Canada over social protection" (Mishra 1990:75). This view is not unanimous. Others (Mullaly 1993; McBride and Shields 1993; Pulkingham and Ternowetsky 1996a) argue that welfare state retrenchment under the Mulroney government is more consequential than Mishra concedes, reflected in a significant erosion of the principle of universality through the clawback of FA, OAS and other policies, in particular the privatization of unemployment insurance.

Perhaps one can equivocate about the impact of neoliberalism in Canada in the 1980s, but the outcome of the 1990s is unequivocal. The fourth offensive to universality came in 1992 with the abandonment of FA and introduction of the Child Tax Benefit (CTB). With this action, the government made absolutely clear its rejection of the principle of universality and the direction in which previous amendments to FA (and arguably, OAS) were headed.

One of the main reasons for implementing the new CTB is to better target low income families with children—a longstanding principle of neoliberalism (Canada 1992; Phipps 1993). In the new CTB, family allowances, the refundable child tax credit and the non-refundable child tax credit are combined into a single "child tax benefit." Two important points are that there is no new money in this package, and parents on welfare (the poorest of the poor) and unemployment insurance receive exactly the same under the new CTB as they did under the previous system.[1] As detailed below, only working parents are eligible for additional benefits from the new CTB.

Families with net incomes under $25,921 get the maximum CTB. After this income threshold, benefit levels are reduced to the point of elimination when income cut-offs are reached for families of different size. The third point is that the income levels at which the CTB is paid are adjusted only when inflation exceeds 3 percent. Between 1992 when the CTB was first announced and the last 1996 federal budget, inflation has remained under 3 percent. As a result many poor families with nominal increases in income "are being pushed above the income threshold for receiving the child tax benefit" (Canadian Council on Social Development [CCSD] 1996a:2). By not indexing the CTB to inflation the federal government cuts out families in need and saves some $160 million a year in CTB payments—a clear example of social policy by stealth that disadvantages those for whom the targeted CTB is purportedly designed (CCSD 1996a:2).

A fourth point about the CTB is that any benefit improvements in this targeted system go only to working poor families, although not all of the working poor benefit (NCW 1992). This preferential treatment stems from the principle of "less eligibility," another tenet of neoliberalism that suggests some poor are "deserving" while others are "undeserving." This principle is embodied in the earned income supplement (later renamed the Working Income Supplement [WIS]), a major new initiative of the CTB when it was first introduced in 1992 by the Conservative government (Canada 1992).

WIS is targeted to the working poor and is not available to individuals in families with children who are not working, whether or not they are in receipt of EI or social assistance. As suggested in William Low's (1996:191) study of financial work incentives provided to welfare mothers, the WIS is based on the premise that people on welfare do not want to work and that incentives are needed to prod them into taking work (see also Phipps 1993).

In the 1996 federal budget, the principle underlying the WIS was entrenched by the Liberals, with increases from the current $500 level to $750 in 1997 and $1000 in 1998 (Department of Supply and Services 1996). While it is important to assist low income families with children in the workforce, the WIS is also a "disciplinary" mechanism (McBride and Shields 1993:34) as it disenfranchises families with children that are not in the workforce. This disenfranchisement is taking place at a time when it is increasingly difficult to find paid employment. Not only is it inappropriate to tie child benefits to a work test but, given the persistence of high unemployment, the WIS disregards the structural circumstances confronting individuals and families with children who are in receipt of EI or social assistance.

An additional issue is that the WIS is also a gendered policy. It penalizes many of the working poor, particularly women, who work part-time and receive low or minimum wages. This occurs as the WIS begins to kick in at an annual wage of $3,750. After $10,000 the full amount of the supplement is paid up to a threshold of $20,921. With high unemployment and the spread of low wage, part-time work, income thresholds of $3,750 and $10,000 may be too high in that they exclude workers earning less. For example, in 1992, when this supplement was first announced, the minimum wage for full-time, full-year work hovered around the $10,000 level in most provinces (Clark 1995:3). This means that part-time workers, many of whom are women with children, would likely be excluded from receiving the full value of the WIS. The WIS not only abandons the poor who are in receipt of EI or social assistance, but it also keeps out the poorest of the working poor. In this respect the CTB fails in its purported intent to better target families with children who are in greatest need.

Despite their lack of popularity among politicians and governments, universal programs are a vital and effective means of supporting children and families. In mapping a way forward, beyond the neoliberal agenda, we need to relearn the value of universality. In part this entails recognizing the failure of targeted programs, such as the CTB, to alleviate poverty. Similar conclusions are reached by several authors (Phipps 1993; Esping-Andersen 1990; McDaniel 1993). For example, Phipps (1993) in her study of child and family benefits under different welfare regimes draws the following conclusions. Income support programs that are targeted to those most in "need" (to achieve the minimal goal of poverty alleviation) are comparatively ineffective as an anti-poverty strategy. Evidence pointing to considerably lower rates of poverty among families with children in European, especially Nordic, countries suggests that pursuit of the "'social democratic' goal of reducing over-all income inequality" is far more effective than the "'liberal' goal of poverty reduction" (Phipps 1993:40). Key to the social democratic model is universal programs and means/income tested programs which provide benefits to the majority of the population (as opposed to means/income tested programs which target benefits only to the extremely "needy") (Phipps 1993:31). In both instances, not only is there less stigma associated with benefit take-up (and therefore greater utilization of programs), programs are much less vulnerable to erosion and elimination because the basis of support is widespread. Finally, the fact is that all universal benefits are conditional (though not income contingent) and target specific groups of beneficiaries. In this way, universal programs are an effective way to target benefits.

Social Safety Net Provisions
As illustrated above, the first line of defence has been abandoned in Canada. During the 1980s and 1990s full employment was gradually redefined as 8 percent unemployment (Department of Finance 1994a; Minister of Supply and Services 1985). Universal programs, such as the family allowance, were replaced by the income tested and targeted child tax benefit (Hess 1992). The universality of OAS was also eliminated, first with the tax clawbacks that began in 1989 and later under the Chrétien government with the new seniors' benefit that is, again, income tested and targeted to those with low income (Department of Finance 1996a).

How about safety net provisions, the second line of defence geared to provide minimum income and services to the poor and most economically disadvantaged? As noted above, Mishra (1990:79) concludes that while these, along with the Canadian welfare state, have been weakened, essentially they remain intact and welfare state continues to be "centrist and evolutionary." This assessment was made in 1990. Six years later it is no longer valid. In particular, the introduction of the CHST has fundamentally weakened the centrist character of the welfare state in Canada.

The impact of the CHST can best be understood by looking at the kind of coverage that is lost with the elimination of CAP (Moscovitch 1996). The first point is that the termination of CAP represents the end of federal legislation that specifically earmarks safety net provisions for the poor and vulnerable. Under CAP approximately two-thirds of federal transfers went to "welfare assistance" and the remainder to "welfare services." The former involves cost shared public (welfare) assistance dollars and the latter, cost shared services that include subsidized daycare to help poor parents enter the workforce, rehabilitative services, counselling and child welfare. The limitations of CAP notwithstanding, its demise in 1996 represents the end of legally mandated services designed to "help lessen, remove or prevent the causes and effect of poverty, child neglect and dependence on public assistance" (Canada 1985:1). A major piece of Canadian legislation, geared to prevent, rehabilitate and alleviate the poverty of the most unprotected, has been cast aside.

A second point is that in contrast to CAP, the CHST's ability to protect those dependent on the safety net is deficient. The CHST is a reduced block fund that combines CAP transfers with those that previously were designated for education and health under the umbrella of established program financing (EPF). In its first two years (1996-97 and 1997-98) total CHST transfers will be some $7 billion less than they would have been had the education, health and CAP transfers remained separate and at their 1995-96 funding levels (Department of Finance 1995). So there is now less money to deal with health and education and safety net demands that, as we noted as the beginning of this chapter, show no signs of subsiding.

A third point is that, as a block fund, the CHST does not designate where final expenditures need to be made (i.e., for education, health or welfare). These decisions are made by the provinces and territories. What the federal government has set up is a situation where dollars traditionally spent on the safety net are now in direct competition with the spending needs of health and education. If we compare the political clout of the health and education sectors with that of welfare, there are grounds for assuming that welfare dollars will be further squeezed as the competition for scarce resources heats up (CCSD 1996b:2).

A fourth point is that, under CAP, provinces had a financial mechanism for responding to growing need as one-half of their additional allocations could be recouped through the 50–50 cost sharing mechanism of CAP.[2] The CHST, in contrast, is not only a reduced fund, but the level of dollars transferred are fixed, and provinces in both good and bad economic times need to make do with their fixed annual allotment. What this ensures is that, in periods of economic decline, there will be fewer federal dollars and therefore less money in total to respond to the growing need for income and related safety net supports.

A fifth point relates to national, minimum standards. Under CAP, safety net expenditures were cost shared by the federal government only if the provinces and territories complied with certain conditions. These included providing assistance to all people judged in need; ensuring benefits levels meet basic needs; not imposing a work requirement as a condition of assistance; setting up an appeal procedure for individuals to challenge welfare decisions; and guaranteeing that residency would not be a requirement of assistance (NCW 1995b; CCSD 1996b:1). Under the CHST only the last condition remains but, as currently witnessed in British Columbia, there are ways to circumvent this and impose a residency requirement as a condition of assistance.[3] When the CHST was first announced these kinds of setbacks were foreshadowed and it was predicted that the elimination of the right to assistance "opens the way for jurisdictions to provide little or no assistance to those in need" (CCSD 1996b:2).

A further point is that, as an instrument of social policy, the CHST constitutes the legislative framework for the devolution of most federal safety net powers to the provinces. It is the backdrop for a decentralized welfare state, where the role of the federal government in terms of setting and enforcing national standards, services and priorities is clearly curtailed (Pawley 1996). CAP provided the legislation and "fiscal carrots" to induce provinces to develop and mount "services for child protection . . . family counseling, rape crises centres, shelters for women and subsidized day care" (CCSD 1996c:5). Over time, depending on the circumstances and political whim of different provinces, these services can now easily disappear. They are no longer mandated by legislation or directly supported by cost shared transfers. The same scenario is applicable to welfare assistance as there is no longer a compulsion to provide assistance to those in need. In 1994 some 3.1 million Canadians received social assistance. Another 1.1 million received help through CAP funded services. Out of these the largest group of recipients were women and children (NCW 1995a:4, 5). Women, as employees and service users/recipients/clients, will be disproportionately impacted by these changes. In particular, low income women will fare worse because they are most likely to rely on social assistance and the many social services that were previously CAP funded, such as daycare subsidies, home care, women's shelters, rape crisis centres and legal aid. As levels of basic protection continue to decline, we can anticipate that those formerly receiving basic assistance from the state will turn, in increasing numbers, to food banks and other non-government agencies for support. A more privatized, residual, neoliberal welfare state seems inevitable as communities, charitable organizations, families and women take on responsibilities formerly assumed by the state (Bach and Rioux 1996).

The CHST is funded through tax points[4] transferred from the federal government to the provinces and a cash transfer. The size of the cash component is declining and is predicted to disappear around 2006 (Battle and Torjman 1996). The concern of the social policy community is that as the cash component declines, so does Ottawa's ability to enforce adherence to the one remaining residency requirement of the CHST (CCSD 1996c).[5] In the February 1996 federal budget a new five year cash floor of $11.1 billion for CHST funding was put in place (Department of Finance 1996b). This new cash floor gives Ottawa the leverage for some provincial compliance, at least until 2003-04. However, by the time this cash floor takes effect (1999-2000), the cash transfers lost to the province since the start of the CHST will reach $7.4 billion. The size of this reduction, in conjunction with the elimination of all but the residency requirement "will likely translate into widespread cuts to programs and supports directed at the most vulnerable Canadians" (Birchall 1996:1). The safety net has been thrown wide open and Ottawa, in its effort to download its financial obligations, is surrendering its role and power to sustain a national system of safety net provisions. The funding levels and limited conditions of the CHST have already set in motion a range of disparate measures of last resort that differ from province to province.

The impact of neoliberalism on safety net provisions is evident in British Columbia's new initiative, BC Benefits. Announced in early 1996, it is designed to ensure support goes to "people truly in need" (Province of British Columbia 1996a:2), a clear neoliberal perspective on the proper role of welfare.

The view that the security provided by welfare is a work disincentive that keeps people from actively seeking employment is also a longstanding, neoliberal critique of the welfare state (McBride and Shields 1993:19). BC Benefits operationalizes these concerns in several ways: it reduces benefit levels for a number of recipients; it denies benefits to those not willing to participate in "active" workfare and learnfare programs; and it disallows benefits to claimants who do not meet the province's new three months residency requirement. Legally, the BC government appears to be able to work around the CHST's residency requirement by redefining welfare as work preparation (Province of British Columbia 1996a). Under CAP this would not have been possible. However, under the vague requirements of the CHST (Remus 1996) the manouverability of the provinces has increased and it seems that there is now room to circumvent the residency requirement.

The denial of benefits to some claimants, across the board reductions for employable recipients and the granting of support "only" if employables participate in workfare and learnfare programs clearly points to an erosion of the safety net. One result of these changes is the reduction in the adequacy of benefits. For employable recipients these now stand at an average of 53 percent of the Statistics Canada poverty line (Ternowetsky 1996).[6] The impact this has on living standards is illustrated by looking at how much income this leaves for food. Entitlement levels in BC are calculated according to two criteria, a shelter and support allowance. For a couple with two children the support allowance now comes to $4.90 per person per day for meals, transportation, clothing, telephone and personal expenses. Indeed it is not surprising that people are turning to charitable, non-government agencies and food banks for help as current levels of assistance are too low on which to get by (Ternowetsky 1996; PG Anti-Poverty Coalition 1996).

Savings from the above changes in rates and eligibility are being used to increase training and workfare opportunities and to fund the new family bonus that provides up to $103 per child (Province of British Columbia 1996b). Ostensibly the family bonus is geared to help families with children. In reality, it is only available to parents who are in the paid labour force. Families with children on social assistance and no member in the paid labour force gain nothing from the family bonus. While they receive it, the entire value is deducted from the support component of the monthly entitlement. This differential treatment of the working poor and unemployed families on social assistance revives the old distinction between the "deserving" and "undeserving" poor, a view of neoliberalism that finds expression in the reduction of safety net provisions for welfare families.

Conclusion

We started the last section by asking "how far down the neoliberal road of welfare state reconstruction have we gone?" The above discussion shows that, in the key policy areas of employment and universal and safety net provisions, the Canadian welfare state has all but collapsed. While there are some signs that the federal government, in conjunction with the provinces and territories, will undertake new national initiatives in the area of child poverty, the nature of these is still unclear. At this time the history of policy developments in the last decade and a half and the current mood of policy restraint, not expansion, suggests this response will be far from adequate. As noted in this chapter the federal government has abandoned its role in key areas of financing, development and maintenance of national programs and standards. In its effort to download fiscal responsibility it has reduced protection for the unemployed in times of high and increasing unemployment; eliminated universal entitlements; and dismantled legislation that once guaranteed minimum safety net provisions across the nation. This retreat is also evident in the federal government's relinquished role among First Nations. The decision not to finance off-reserve costs for social assistance leaves First Nations people even more vulnerable.

What these developments imply is that, in the face of growing economic insecurity, the state will continue to assume less and less responsibility for the collective well-being of its citizenry. In the areas of employment and universal and safety net measures, the welfare state is being reduced to a residual role of last resort. But even in this context, benefit levels and entitlements are so low and unpredictable that basic needs are increasingly being met by charitable organizations, the family and a weakened non-government sector. For social policy in general, and child and family policies in particular, the future is one of a growing minimalist welfare state that will do little to reverse the widespread economic vulnerability of the people who live and work in this country.

Notes

1. Under this new system of child benefits, the equivalent to married credit and the childcare deduction remain intact, although the value of the childcare deduction was increased by the Conservatives when the plan was first introduced and again later by the Liberals. The childcare deduction is a regressive tax measure. It reduces the tax paid for middle and upper income earners, but provides no benefit to poor families with children that do not pay tax. In the same way, the equivalent to married credit in a lone parent family treats the oldest child as a spouse and provides a tax credit equal to the spousal deduction. Once again, this assists only lone parents who earn enough money to pay taxes.

2. In 1990 this 50–50 formula changed for the three richest provinces: Ontario, Alberta and British Columbia. After 1990 a cap on annual CAP transfers was set at 5 percent increases for these provinces. This had the effect of substantially reducing the federal share of welfare expenditures made by these provinces (NCW 1995b:7).

3. When the BC government first imposed a residency requirement in 1996 the federal

government challenged this in the courts. However, the BC government appears to have circumvented this requirement by passing BC Benefits, a new system that redefines welfare as training.

4. Tax point transfers are "a reduction of federal tax rates allowing provinces to raise additional revenues without increasing the overall tax burden" (Department of Finance 1996b:1).

5. There is a similar concern that enforcement of the standards of the Canada Health Act will be compromised.

6. This is for a mid-sized city with a population between 60,000 and 99,000. Except for singles and couples without children, the situation is worse for unemployable families with children. They receive on average about 45 percent of Statistics Canada's low income measure of adequacy (PG Anti-Poverty Coalition 1996).

Part 2:
Feminist and First Nations Critiques of Child Welfare

Victims and Villains: Scandals, the Press and Policy Making in Child Welfare

MARILYN CALLAHAN AND KAREN CALLAHAN

"Death has the advantage of being unambiguous, producing both victim and villain" (Aldridge 1990:616).

Introduction

There is ample evidence that the press is uninterested in child welfare, until a tragedy occurs (Franklin and Parton 1991). When parents kill or injure their child or a childcare agency fails children in its care, or both, then the press coverage is often unremitting. Press stories about these misfortunes are garnered from disaffected friends or neighbours or coroners' reports, while those most directly involved are silent: the parents because of their shame and possible criminal charges; the workers, managers and politicians because of policies of confidentiality.

The purpose of this paper is to examine press coverage of a public inquiry of a child welfare tragedy and compare it to the actual testimony given at the inquiry. The specific case involved the death of Matthew Vaudreuil in British Columbia, the subsequent sentencing of his mother for the offence and a public inquiry into the circumstances after the trial. We view the news "not [as] a picture of reality which may be correct or biased, but as a frame through which the social world is routinely constructed" (Van Dijk 1993:7-8). We wanted to know what reporters chose to report, what reality they attempted to construct and how they did it. What makes this case particularly interesting is the fact that verbatim transcripts of the events in questions are available. The power of the press is partly obtained by its ability to make us "indirect witnesses to events of which we have no first-hand knowledge or experience" (Bennett 1982). What do we learn when we can compare a full record with press reports? Do reporters, having access to a great deal of information about child welfare, as they did about this particular case, write different stories than reporters who have fewer informants?[1]

Unravelling the images of child welfare and social workers that are created in the press is a meaningful task. At a time when all social programs are under scrutiny, it is vital to examine how the press portrays the very people and programs who will be affected by proposed cuts to social spending. The child welfare cases most likely to be given intense media scrutiny are the unusual ones: the Vaudreuil case was uncommon because a mother killed her child, much like the Susan Smith situation in the U.S. where the guilty mother was featured on the front page of *Time* (1994). The selection of unusual cases for scrutiny, while ignoring or diminishing routine situations, distorts public perceptions. Women, particularly poor single women, are seen to be doing a bad job of looking after children. Welfare bashing of single parent women has become common in the U.S. and parts of Canada and sensational child welfare stories feed the myths of women on welfare. Social work students and practitioners are often dispirited by media coverage of their work (Callahan 1994). While they vehemently dispute media versions of their actions, they feel at a loss to correct such stories. Policy makers, particularly politicians, respond hastily to unfavourable press coverage in child welfare as they wish to be on the side of children and justice. Thus we often have "policy making by panic," resulting in even more rules and regulations for harried workers.

The Approach to Analysis

We limited our study to press coverage only, given the difficulty of capturing television and radio news retrospectively. We also limited our inquiry to the coverage in *The Vancouver Sun* as it is the major newspaper in British Columbia and claims a reputation of a fair minded mainstream press. We have examined press coverage of the case throughout its duration but will highlight one period only, from August to December 1994 during the initial stages of the judicial inquiry into the death of Matthew Vaudreuil. This phase was selected because it includes rich testimony from a panoply of characters in child welfare and, pragmatically, because transcripts for this segment of the inquiry were available.

We used two approaches to analyzing our data. The first involved a content analysis of all of the stories which were then categorized on the basis of the following: theme, length (column inches), location (first page, feature page, back page), original story or Canadian Press story, author (editorial, by-line general story) and sources of information for the story (clients, social workers, administrators, politicians, outside experts, others).[2]

The second, critical discourse analysis based primarily on the work of Van Dijk (1988), focused upon the use of words, patterns and structures to reinforce prevailing discourses. Critical discourse analysis draws attention to several features of text. One, *macrostructural* analysis, suggests that readers tend to derive meaning from texts according to the knowledge they already possess about the world (Van Dijk 1988:13-14). Members of a single culture generally share knowledge about certain events—for example, about what it means to "go for a drive" or to "graduate from high school"—and therefore often draw on similar information in the interpretation of texts.

Another, *intertextual* analysis, examines the relationship among central messages. As readers tend to remember only the headline and the first paragraph of newspaper stories, these effectively form the summary of the information contained below them, and present readers with a convenient thematic precis, ready-made for commission to memory. When a series of stories on the same topic appear in a given newspaper, the theme of that series is set by the headline and first paragraph of the first story. For those readers who follow the whole series from beginning to end, all information which follows will be interpreted in the context of the initial theme. We read instalments of a story not in a vacuum, but with reference to each other. The third ingredient, *grammatical* analysis, investigates how these themes are invoked and reproduced at the level of the sentence. Three main grammatical features of press accounts are important for the analysis of our stories: the inverted declarative sentence; the use of passive and active voice; and relational functions (Van Dijk 1988:11).

Relevance structuring refers to the simple principle that the most important information in a news text is stated first. Whole stories can be examined in terms of relevance structuring. Although the headline and lead paragraph of news accounts summarize what is implicitly the most important aspect of the story, relevance structuring also applies at the level of the sentence. The information given at the beginning of the sentence is implicitly more significant than that left to the end. Finally, the term *rhetorical structures* refers to a variety of strategies employed at all levels to make the text more persuasive. News reports may use techniques such as repetition, rhyme or assonance, hyperbole or understatement, sharply contrasting images and words and sentences which build a climax. For example, Barthes (1988:172) states that the posing of an enigma represents a well worn climax-building strategy. Enigmatic titles or headlines serve an aperitive function: that is, they whet the readers' appetites, suggesting that a solution rests somewhere in the text which follows.

The Findings in a Nutshell:
The Story of Victims and Villains

After examining literally thousands of pages of transcripts and hundreds of articles, we have come to a simple conclusion. The very first article written about the case, at the sentencing of the mother for the death and long before the public inquiry began, set the tone for all that followed.[3] The story told in the press is one of an evil mother who cared more for herself, her boyfriends and her seedy lifestyle than for her child. According to this account, many social workers knew about the mother's wholly inadequate care but did nothing about it. Extended family members and friends urged social workers to intervene but workers still did nothing, insulting and dismissing those who tried to help. When the child died, social workers tried to cover up their ineffectiveness by changing case records. Even the top child welfare worker in the province, the superintendent of child welfare, was portrayed as having altered a report on the child's death, putting her ministry in a much more favourable light with her changes.

The press stories maintain that social workers behaved in this fashion because they are simple-minded and easily duped by a deceitful mother. They think that they can assess character but they are really very incompetent. They also ignored obvious signs of child abuse and neglect because the government had changed policy, making it easier for an inadequate mother to keep her child. Social workers do not have the courage to defy government policies, even when they have plenty of evidence to the contrary. However, when given a bit of power, social workers push around those whom they can in an effort to ensure that their own interests are protected at all costs.

The story told in the transcripts is considerably more complex. Here we see a mother who was sometimes inadequate, sometimes capable, sometimes neglectful, sometimes very loving. We have a picture of a mother who was abused and neglected by her own father and who spent most of her life in care. She is described as being mentally handicapped and living her life on a marginal income. We see friends whose testimony was inconsistent and contradictory and few family members who supported her overall. We also encounter a mother who may have neglected her child to the point of his death. This last point is even unclear.

The story of social services and social work practice in the transcripts is also much more complicated. We have examples of social workers taking prudent actions to investigate complaints, mounting thousands of dollars of support services to the family and taking considerable time and attention to help the mother and child. There is no evidence that documents were changed to cover up any wrongdoing. Even the alleged alteration of the report by the superintendent of child welfare is refuted by those who wrote earlier drafts of that report and others who reviewed it prior to its release. However, in the end, we have a child that died and many actions that could have been taken to prevent his death.

We have one final conclusion: that having access to vast amounts of information *in this case at least* did not change the way these reporters covered a sensational child welfare case. The same themes and images portrayed in this case were evident in the research by Franklin and Parton (1991) who suggest that two specific types of child abuse "stories" receive the most extensive coverage in the mainstream media: the case where the social worker intervenes unsuccessfully in the family and the child is injured or murdered; and the situation where workers remove children from parents and the decision is reversed, often by the court. These authors identify two unfavourable and contradictory images of social workers. One is the stereotype of social workers as "wimps": incompetent, non-judgmental and indecisive, behaving as "butterflies in . . . situation[s] that demand hawks" (Franklin and Parton 1991:273). They are as guilty for the death of the abused child as the abuser. As a result, social work "wimps" are often simultaneously labelled as "killers" of children.

By contrast, the second type of child abuse story produces an image of social workers as "authoritarian bureaucrats," "empire builders" and "abusers of authority," in short as "bullies." Winter (1992) argues, after an examination of the Cleveland affair in Britain, that the press portrayed social workers as exaggerating sexual abuse claims in order to retain their jobs and their authority.

While previous research indicates that one or the other of these images is contained in a particular story of child abuse, the coverage of social workers in the Vaudreuil case contained both of these stereotypes and even a third, the "charlatan." As "wimps," social workers are featured time and again throughout the press stories as failing to act promptly and decisively for Matthew's benefit and, instead, believing the insincere and transparent blandishments of the mother. The "bully" image is constructed not on the basis of social workers acting precipitously and removing children unnecessarily, but through their refusal to share important information with other helpers and their cavalier treatment of apparently helpful and caring family members. As "charlatans," social workers supposedly tried to cover up their incompetence as "wimps and bullies" by not informing others of important facts which could have saved the child. In addition, they supposedly doctored records to save their own reputations after Matthew's death and provided vague and self-serving testimony at the inquiry. It is hard to imagine more damaging images to social workers than the combination of these three images. Not only are social workers portrayed in the press as ineffectual at their job, they oppress those beneath them and care more about themselves than they do about obtaining justice for a murdered child.

An Example of Press Coverage and Transcriptions

The next section of this chapter examines how reporters created villains and victims by consistently distorting or eliminating any evidence which refuted their conclusions. Given the overwhelming numbers of stories and the volume of transcripts, we have selected only one to illustrate how reporters accomplished their purposes. The following selection was chosen after a careful examination of fifty-nine press stories in *The Vancouver Sun* and all transcripts from August to December, 1994. The story fits the typical profile of all stories in terms of length, placement in the paper and author (one of the principal reporters covering the case).

The story in *The Vancouver Sun* on September 14 (Cannata 1994:B3) begins with the headline and sub-heading: "Two faces of child killer: sweet, then bitter"; "Vaudreuil's personality dissected." The term, "two faces," the first and thus most privileged information in this article, establishes the theme by drawing on cultural scripts about "good" and "bad" women and female duplicity. There are two types of women in the world, the well worn script reads: some are "good" (that is, selfless, innocuous and chaste) and others are simply "bad" (that is, selfish, dangerous and promiscuous). Another script (which has endured for centuries in Western discourse and which has become increasingly popular over the last decade) casts women as inherently duplicitous or "two-faced" (Faludi 1991:116). Duplicitous women appear "good" on the outside when, in fact, they are wholly evil on the inside.

Ania Wilczynski (1991) has demonstrated the current prominence of this construction of "woman" in her examination of women charged with killing their own children. They are either constructed by the press and the justice system as insane or, more commonly, as evil. Bad women are "viewed as ruthless, selfish, cold, callous, neglectful of their children or domestic responsibilities, violent or promiscuous" (Wilczynski 1991:76). The explanation of their crimes need go no farther than the invocation of this well worn theme: the woman in question killed, we understand, simply because she was bad (Wilczynski 1991). In their study of convictions of mothers who kill their children, Morris and Wilczynski (1994) noted that those mothers who appear contrite and cowed by the experience are more likely to be judged "insane," while those who seem defiant or enigmatic are more likely to be branded "bad."

The use of the phrase "child killer" serves to reinforce the cultural scripts invoked by the words "two faces." In case there was any doubt about which "type" of woman readers will encounter in the body of the article, the words "child killer" confirm her status as a "bad" woman. Note also that the phrase "child killer" is ambiguous. It could refer to one child or many children. Vaudreuil is again associated with other criminals for whom the term "child killer" applies—among them, vicious serial killers (as she was at the beginning of the press coverage of this story). In the first five words of the headline, readers are given the (implicitly most significant) information that the subject of the article is a woman who not only pretends to be good to camouflage her true, evil self, but who is also a murderer of children. The woman, Verna Vaudreuil, is identified by name in the subheading. In terms of relevance structuring, this word order ensures that the reader knows that she is a child killer first and foremost.

Following the colon, the words "sweet, then bitter" clarify and reinforce the initial phrase "two faces." We can identify the rhetorical use of contrast here: the binary opposition "sweet/bitter" emphasizes the "good/bad" opposition invoked at the beginning of the sentence. Rhetorically, the use of binary opposition serves to persuade the reader that the character in question had two distinct, opposing facets to her personality. She was sweet, then bitter; apparently good, but actually bad. These oppositions close the door on any further investigation into the nature of Vaudreuil's personality and leave no room for any discussion of "grey areas" or complexity. The body of the article which, the subheading promises, "dissect[s]" Vaudreuil's personality, will be read in terms of the dualism established by the headline.

The subheading "Vaudreuil's personality dissected" calls up a third cultural script about scientific investigation. The word "dissect" refers to a scientific (and hence, objective) delving below the surface to "discover" the "truth" of whatever lies below. According to the script of scientific investigation, the article which follows the headline will uncover the real facts of this case and, in particular, it will unveil Vaudreuil's "true" self. Further, these two phrases imply that there is a secret to Vaudreuil's personality which will be at least partly disclosed in the body of the article. The use of the phrase "two faces" works to hint at the solution and thus to intensify the aperitive effect.

The grammatical structure of these two headings reinforces their messages. The information contained in the headline summarizes direct quotes from the body of the article, yet in the headline no speaker is identified and no quotation marks are used. The implication is that these words do not represent one (potentially biased) person's opinion, but rather they describe the objective "truth" of Vaudreuil's personality. The invocation of a scientific script, as already mentioned, underscores this message. Grammatically, the headline bears no resemblance to the standard subject + verb + object sentence structure. Instead it consists of two descriptive phrases: "two faces of child killer" and "sweet, then bitter." What is missing before the words "two faces" is the identity of the subject of the sentence: "witness describes two faces of child killer." This is an example of complete sentence alternatives to the incomplete structure used in the headline. Again, the identity of the speaker is effectively buried through the use of this grammatical structure. Similarly, the passive voice is used in the subheading, which reads "Vaudreuil's personality dissected" rather than "witnesses dissect Vaudreuil's personality." Although "Vaudreuil" is still the object of the sentence, she is cast in the subject position, thus emphasizing her agency and hence culpability in this crime. This grammatical structure also masks the identity of exactly who is doing the "dissect[ing]" of Vaudreuil's personality. Given that the word "dissect" activates a scientific script, the implication is that Vaudreuil has been subjected to a fair and unbiased psychological evaluation by some kind of expert. Completely different ideological implications would flow from a heading which read "Friend gives opinion on Vaudreuil's personality." Masking the friend's identity works to invest the results of the personality dissection with scientific authority, and hence to render the "two faces" diagnosis objective, "true" and final.

The first, single-sentence paragraph of the article reads: "She showed one face to the public and a vastly different side of herself to the people who knew her." Once again, while this information summarizes the spoken words of a couple of witnesses, we find no quotation marks, no speaker identified. The statement is simply presented as "true." Thematically, this sentence reinscribes the theme of duplicity set out in the headline: Vaudreuil had "one [good] face" and a "vastly different [evil] side." Grammatically, "she" (Vaudreuil) is placed in the subject position of the sentence, highlighting her status as agent. Casting Vaudreuil as the subject of the sentence, together with the use of the verb "showed," further emphasizes her duplicity: Vaudreuil *deliberately* constructed an innocent appearance, this grammatical structure implies, in order to further her own evil designs. And again, we note the rhetorical use of dualism: Vaudreuil had two distinct and opposing sides to her personality, this paragraph reminds us, and no more.

46

The second paragraph continues: "And if you talked to her about it, as her cousin Lynnette Milligan once did, she'd tell you she regretted having a son and wouldn't if she had to do it again." This paragraph serves to clarify paragraph one and sustain the theme set out in the headline, providing, implicitly, a specific example of Vaudreuil showing "a vastly different side of herself to the people who knew her." We already know that Vaudreuil has "two faces" and that she showed the "bad" side to the people she knew well, so that this admission of regret to her cousin must be an illustration of her true, hidden, evil self. We note a fourth cultural script. This is about motherhood and specifically about what it means to be a good mother. Good mothers are selflessly and completely devoted to ensuring the happiness and well-being of their children. They are fulfilled by, and grateful for, the experience of motherhood. They are not ambivalent and certainly not regretful about it. We should also note that the use of the conditional tense obscures the fact that Vaudreuil expressed regret to her cousin on one occasion only. We are told, instead, that Vaudreuil *would* express regret. This use of the conditional verb tense implies that Vaudreuil complained repeatedly and frequently in the past about her dissatisfaction with motherhood. Finally, while this paragraph again summarizes the words of one witness, there is still no speaker identified. Rather, the emphasis here is on Vaudreuil's past speech.

Paragraph three states: "That was the glimpse people got into the life of Verna Vaudreuil Tuesday at the Gove Inquiry into child protection, now in its third week." Here again, the passive voice is used to mask the identity of the person who provided the "glimpse" into Vaudreuil's life. This use of the passive suggests that the glimpse people got was into Vaudreuil's *real* life—as through the window of her house or the lens of a telescope—and not into some individual's (necessarily partial) *version* of that life. Furthermore, the use of the word "glimpse" sustains the scientific motif invoked by the headline: we are looking into Vaudreuil's past, this word suggests, delving below her innocent exterior, "dis-covering" the (buried) truth.

Paragraph four continues: "Vaudreuil is serving 10 years in prison after admitting she suffocated Matthew, then 5, in 1992 by placing her hand over his nose and mouth to try to discipline him." The common rhetorical strategy of excessive use of numbers, implying precision and objectivity, is used again. The rhetorical use of repetition is apparent in this paragraph as well: in one sentence, we are told both that Vaudreuil "suffocated" her son and that she "plac[ed] her hand over his nose and mouth." This repetition serves to place a great deal of emphasis on exactly how Vaudreuil killed her child. Moreover, the grammatical structure of the sentence underscores Vaudreuil's agency: not only is "Vaudreuil" in the subject position of the sentence, she is also described as performing various actions throughout. She is *serving* 10 years after *admitting* she *suffocated* Matthew by *placing* her hand over his nose and mouth to *discipline* him.

Paragraph five: "She is mentally handicapped, has a history of involvement with the social services ministry and suffered abuse herself as a child." The content of this paragraph seems to be working against the "evil/duplicitous" woman theme as it states that Vaudreuil herself was a victim of abuse. But if we look at how this information is stated, we can begin to see that the grammar of this sentence works in effect to dismiss its content. Vaudreuil is still in the subject position in this sentence. The identity of the people who abused her is buried. No one does anything *to* Vaudreuil here; rather she remains the subject throughout and bad things appear to just "happen" to her as the result of nothing but ill luck. Note also the lack of detail here: all we are told is that Vaudreuil "has a history of involvement" with social services and that she "suffered" some kind of abuse. Compare this sentence with the numerous sentences describing Vaudreuil's abuse of her child. The overall effect, we would argue, is to dismiss Vaudreuil's childhood experiences of abuse as any kind of explanation for her crime. What happened to her is minimized, while what she did to her child is emphasized again and again. Note that very different ideological implications would flow from an article that devoted half of its column inches to descriptions of the specific abuse Verna Vaudreuil suffered as a child.

Paragraphs six to twenty-two contain either direct quotes by or the reported speech of two witnesses: Lynette Milligan, Vaudreuil's cousin, and Kathy Masse, a friend. Milligan and Masse give examples illustrating Vaudreuil's "two-faced" personality and deliberate duplicity. Since we are told at the beginning of the article that Vaudreuil showed her evil side to the people she knew well, and since these two women apparently knew Vaudreuil, their statements are invested with authority. In paragraphs seventeen and nineteen, Milligan describes Vaudreuil as actively covering up the truth of her abusive behaviour.

The transcripts of the day in question in this press story tell quite a different story about the mother. In her testimony Lynette Milligan reported that when she first began visiting Vaudreuil, the house was reasonably tidy, Matthew had a lot of toys and there was some affection between mother and child. "He'd go over and give her a hug or kiss" (*Gove Inquiry* 1994a:1701). Verna would play with Matthew and Matthew's behaviour was "average" (1702). During the time that Lynette lived with Verna and Matthew, when Matthew was about three years old, she described Verna as providing breakfast and walking him to and from his playschool, making sure that he was in bed regularly by 8:00 pm and that no one else slept in his room. She responded to Matthew's tantrums by telling him to go to his room. She also punished him verbally saying "No, that's wrong, you shouldn't do that" and "You can't do that," and then "He'd go into his tantrum and beat himself up." Milligan never saw Verna hit Matthew nor did she ever hear her wish that Matthew would be taken away in the two months she lived with them. Some of the dialogue provides the flavour of her testimony:

Q. Did you have concerns for Matthew?

A. Not real life-threatening concerns, no.

Q. Do you think Verna loved Matthew?

A. In her own way, yes.

A. Did you think she was a good mother to Matthew.

A. Sometimes yes.

Q. And the other times?

A. I thought she was a little bit too hard on him. (*Gove Inquiry* 1994a:1733).

In response to concerns about her potential for violence, Milligan states: "No. She would get to the point where you could just see that she was—getting to the point where she was going to lose it, and then she'd just calm right down" (1742).

Two other witnesses, Kathy Masse and Tina Calder, also testified about Vaudreuil's treatment of her child. Calder told of occasions when Verna apparently "kicked Matthew and threw him up against the wall." Both recounted another occasion where they heard someone say that Matthew had been burned on his penis, an incident which Masse states she reported to social services, although she did not see evidence of it herself. Interestingly, these rather sensational although dubious facts were scarcely reported in the story. (Tina Calder was not mentioned at all in the press story which may be explained because she testified last in the day and reporters may have left to file their stories.) Instead, the attempts by Masse to contact social services (over sixty calls) were included in the press story. However, none of the evidence contradicting this testimony was included. For instance counsel (McHale) for the Ministry of Social Services stated that records showed Masse contacting the ministry only two or three times. The testimony that she did not report any of these complaints in person, did not have a phone during this period and had reasons to dislike Verna Vaudreuil was not reported. Most importantly the press account omitted the fact that at least one of the reports was followed up by a visit from the social worker and an examination by a physician and found unsubstantiated.

Altogether, the testimony about the mother's treatment of the child on this particular day bears little resemblance to the press story. Instead, we are introduced to a mother who seemed to have had periods of caring well for her child and was, at worst, sometimes impatient. Only one witness actually saw the mother harm the child, although not seriously enough to report it.

Social workers are described in paragraphs twenty-four to twenty-eight of the press story (Cannata 1994:B3) as covering up the truth of Vaudreuil's situation: "social services staff kept home support workers in the dark about details of Vaudreuil's problems when they were contracted to work in her home, the inquiry also heard on Tuesday." The rhetorical device of parallelism used here has the effect of suggesting a clear similarity between Vaudreuil's behaviour, "two-faced" and duplicitous, and that of the social workers involved. Implicitly, then, the social workers are just as culpable for Matthew's death as is Vaudreuil.

In support of this proposition, the press quoted Fran Roach, a homemaker who had worked with Ms. Vaudreuil and Matthew:

> "We could certainly provide a much better service, be able to pick out the right person if we know the particulars," Roach said. . . . For example, Roach said she had no idea ministry staff were considering apprehending Matthew in 1989 if conditions in his household didn't improve.

In fact, the press story ends on this note, implying that this information could have made a great deal of difference to the homemakers and helped Matthew as well. However, testimony in the transcripts provides a different picture. Roach did, at one point, regret that confidentiality policies often impeded their placing the most appropriate homemaker. The dialogue continues however:

> Q. And did you know . . . that the social worker . . . had serious concerns about Verna's ability to parent Matthew and was considering apprehension as a possibility?
> A. Was considering apprehension? No I did not know that.

Here is where the press story ends; however, the testimony continues:

> Q. If you had known that—that those kinds of concerns existed and that was being considered—apprehension was being considered as a possibility, would that have been helpful to you in reporting back to your contract?
> A. It might have, *except I think we did*—I know over the years with Verna and Matthew, I talked to people at Social Services a lot, you know. . . . *(Gove Inquiry* 1994a:1679; emphasis added)

According to the press account, the reasons that social workers do not tell homemakers and others about the helpful particulars of any case is stated as follows: "But ministry rules about client confidentiality often mean contract workers like homemakers don't get all the client's history beforehand." Social workers appear to be thoughtlessly following "rules" that hinder good childcare and respectful work with other colleagues. However, at the inquiry, Anne Dunfield, the administrator of the North Peace Home Support Services testified that her organization also had a policy of confidentiality, much like that of social services. The reason for this policy was that the society, which hired young, often inexperienced workers, did not want "people talking to their neighbours or their friends about their clients or about their work situations" *(Gove Inquiry* 1994a:1641). While confidentiality is portrayed as a hindrance in the press account, good reasons for its existence are provided in the transcripts.

Dunfield further stated that the agency had a policy enabling home support workers to report important information about their clients to Social Services. The homemakers in the home for a two month period recorded dirty conditions and behaviour problems with Matthew but did not record or report concerns about neglect or abuse. This information was not included in the press story.

The intent of this section of the chapter is to demonstrate how the press accounts of the public inquiry highlighted only testimony which supported the original themes of the story, set long before the inquiry began, and distorted or eliminated testimony which provided contradictory information. Thus readers were not expected to understand the complexity of the situation, grapple with the fact that mothers can be both caring and neglectful and that workers can be both careful and yet overlook important information. They were not expected to deal with the context of the lives of mothers and workers, a mother with few resources unable to cope with the day-to-day care of a child and workers who testified as this one did:

> I think it is important to understand that social workers work in the context. Sometimes I get the impression that the public . . . think that we work in a library where information is readily available, where it's categorized and so on, but the world of a protection social worker isn't like that, it's not that neat and clean. We have to work under a lot of pressure. We work high caseloads. We work in the situation where the facts . . . are always kind of floating, they're always changing colour and where decisions have to be made on sometimes sketchy information and frankly where some people lie to you. . . . There's a social context in which we work where clearly, if one reads the newspapers and watches the media, half the population thinks we intervene too much and the other half thinks we don't intervene enough and it's under those kind of conditions and those kind of pressures that social workers are trying to do their job. . . . *(Gove Inquiry* 1994b:227)

Instead, the editor of the paper, Ian Haysom, wrote another editorial at the end of days of conflicting testimony about mothers and workers. Unflinching from his original theme set in his editorials six months previously, he stated:

> There is no describing the horror of a case in which a little boy was tortured by his own mother for five years and finally killed. But the best hope of preventing a recurrence is that someone take responsibility and fix the system. If the New Democrats go on trying to blame someone else, there is little hope for improvement. (1994:A24)

Why the Paper Chose to Report the Story as It Did

Many reasons have been proposed for the press interest in dramatic child abuse stories (Franklin and Parton 1991). They make good copy and meet the criteria of "good stories," those which are based upon "human interest, life and death, sex and conflict" (Fry 1991:66). Wroe (1988:20-24) expands upon Fry's analysis, using Chibnall's (1977) standard list of "eight imperatives controlling journalism"—immediacy, dramatization, personalization, simplification, titillation, conventionalism, structured access and novelty—to explain the over-reporting of social work/child abuse stories in the British press. For Wroe, the typical child abuse stories fit neatly into established news patterns. For instance, while much day-to-day social work practice is "slow and indeterminate, the death of a child is an exception" and an immediate, definable event. It is dramatic and lends itself to the "vocabulary of dramatic conflict" (Wroe 1988:44). Moreover, the child abuse story translates well into a conventional news story with "familiar scenarios, cliches, images and stereotypes" and is thus "rendered immediately intelligible" (Wroe 1988:44). The pattern of child abuse cases includes an unfolding narrative which can be continued day after day from the trial, to the revelation of social services inadequacies, the search for someone to blame, the public inquiry and finally the publication of the inquiry report.

In this case there was an innocent child killed by his mother: the mother killer was unrepentant; police prosecutors and defence "cut a deal" which the judge overruled; relatives and friends complained to no avail; incompetent social workers ignored obvious signs of abuse; and the government changed its policies to "go softer" on errant mothers. The press can appear to side with the innocent and powerless, a child and his poor-but-well-meaning relatives who are defenceless against uncaring bureaucrats and misbegotten government policies. It speaks to the powerlessness that many readers feel and at the same time offers assurance to these same readers that the press is on their side, all the while offering them a titillating story written as a serialized morality play. As businesses in themselves, newspapers have to be concerned about what sells; stories about "some worthy policy development practice initiative or social services personality are never published simply because there is no market for them" (Wroe 1988:67; Herman and Chomsky 1988).

While the explanation of child abuse as "good copy" is useful, Hachey and Grenier argue that child abuse, told as personal, immediate stories in the press, is the result of the "dominant capitalist ideology operating upon and through mass media representations" (1992:236). The media's emphasis on "individual rather than structural causes diverts attention away from the structure of power relations in capitalist society" (Hachey and Grenier 1992:236). For instance, blaming mothers or individual social workers for a child's death ends the story, rendering further discussion and analysis unnecessary. The status quo is reaffirmed: social structures require few changes; the behaviour of people who deviate from prescribed norms "is an expression of their differentness, their sad inability to live by the sensible rules of normal society" (Chibnall 1977:20).

In this case Verna Vaudreuil can be vilified because she apparently forsook the help and support of her extended family, insisted on living with a series of undesirable men rather than marry a caring father for the child, and indulged in disreputable behaviour well beyond the pale of ordinary women. In spite of the evidence that the family abused Vaudreuil from the time she was a child, that the child's father was in jail most of the time and offered no support to Vaudreuil or the child and that there was no substantiated evidence of excessive drinking, drugs or prostitution, Verna Vaudreuil stands as a woman who shunned the succour of the family and thus deserved her fate.

The messages about state intervention in families in this case are more subtle. On the one hand, those favouring family values might cheer social workers who worked to protect parental rights and strengthen Verna's family. However, time and again in the press coverage we are reminded that this particular family, Verna, Matthew and assorted boyfriends, was not a properly constituted one and thus should not have been preserved. The amount of press coverage given to the highly questionable statements by Vaudreuil's family about its desire to care for Matthew suggests that social workers should have broken up a single-parent family and strengthened the properly constituted extended family of aunts, fathers and grandfathers. In the end, the press account does not support state intervention in families nor state care for children; instead it supports state action to dissolve improper families and support traditional ones.

Franklin and Parton (1991) have developed this argument further in explaining why social workers are continually vilified for their handling of child welfare cases. Social work as a profession provides services previously offered within families and communities: caring, counselling and problem solving. Professionalizing these services "offers an implicit critique of the family and community": that is, if families and communities are functioning as they should, there should be no need for social workers (Franklin and Parton 1991:9). By its very existence, then, the profession of social work suggests that the heterosexual nuclear family—often called the basic building block of society—is essentially unstable and unworkable or, at the very least, in need of state assistance in order to function (Winter 1992:9). Therefore finding fault with the performance of individual social workers calls into question the value and necessity of the profession overall and reaffirms the capabilities of family and community. Thus child welfare tragedies provide fertile material for press stories and it is no wonder that they are featured. They meet all of the criteria for a good story and they serve to bolster dominant cultural values about families, women and state responsibility for social issues while reinforcing the neutrality of the press. Perhaps in present day uncertainties, they provide a cultural script of a "simpler" time that is long past and that soothes all of us—workers, clients, readers and reporters. As an old detective once said: "Life would be a great deal easier at times, if we could like all the heroes and dislike all the villains. Or personally,

I'd settle for simply not pitying the villains as much as I do the victims half the time" (Perry 1991:315-16).

What the Press Missed

Everywhere in the transcripts are avenues for inquiry completely missed by the press, intent as they were on portraying a child victim, a villainous mother and incompetent workers. Several threads are missing. There is little mention of the numbers of largely uncoordinated services which one mother must expect to manage nor of the short term nature of most of these services, built as they are on a model of social learning and not on one of long term social support. Nor does the press focus upon a compelling story for investigative journalism concerning what actually happened to Matthew and who killed him, uncertain as facts are concerning the perpetrator of the crime and the actions of the mother and her last boyfriend in the final weeks of the child's life.

Consider one of these angles: uncoordinated services. During an eight month period, the Ministry of Social Services, the public child welfare agency, provided the family with no less than five workers: one social worker to carry out a protection investigation who referred the family to a worker for mentally handicapped services and two family service workers who mobilized a range of family services. Further, a financial assistance worker assessed their eligibility for welfare and referred them to mental health services because of past traumas. The family service workers in turn contracted with a number of community agencies to provide a special needs daycare and assessment centre; a home-maker service; a childcare service; a parenting program and a foster mother for respite care. Other community agencies became involved. The transition house and second stage housing societies provided accommodation and programs, the police were contacted around possible abuse by the husband and the food bank and victim support services offered other resources.

In the midst of all of this was a mother with modest intellectual and coping abilities and a child who had been moved several times, cared for by many different people and with little certainty in his short life. There were workers with high caseloads, some new on the job, who rarely spoke to one another. They had little time to sit down with the mother, tell her how they differed from the plethora of other workers and sort out plans.

Why have these particular child welfare services become so fractured with four separate offices having differing functions and specializations? How can families understand this organization? The standard response to these questions is that more coordination of services is required and that social workers should assume the role of case managers. Reporters could have inquired whether the culture of referral evident in this case would continue to exist under case management systems. They could have asked whether the time spent by one skilled worker doing many of the above jobs would not have resulted in a far more effective assessment at much less cost to child, mother, worker and taxpayer. Following these threads would have been no less kind to government or to social workers but may have made a difference to child welfare. Only glimmers of these insights appeared occasionally in the coverage of this story (Cannata 1994:B3), usually at the end of the feature.

Influencing the Press

We began this study curious about whether having access to a great deal of information about a particular child welfare tragedy would influence the way reporters wrote about the case. Clearly it did not. The same patterns as noted by Franklin and Parton (1991) in their analysis of the British coverage of child welfare were evident in this case study.

These findings should give social workers and other activists pause for reflection. The strategy of trying to combat press stories of child welfare with more facts may be doomed from the beginning, given other powerful forces: making money, political warmongering and settling ideological disputes which encourage the press to cover child welfare as it does already.

Someone once said that "any press is better than no press." In September 1995 two hundred and fifty new social work positions were created in child welfare in B.C., most certainly because of this particular situation. Some might argue that the only way child welfare will gain resources is through publicity of the sort it received during this case. It is an insufficiently important item on the social welfare agenda to command the time of policy makers without pressure, however negative, from the press.

We are not convinced that this is a sound argument, primarily because negative press can also lead to more stringent policies and procedures, making child welfare work even more impossible. Instead, we think that social workers should analyze press coverage and find ways to expose others to media bias and misinformation. This article is one attempt. The analysis by Aldridge (1990) is also persuasive. She states that we should never underestimate the power of profit in the press. Unless we are willing to abandon our principles and portray ourselves as "social police" or give up our social analysis and talk only of "titillating personal problems" our stories will have little currency.

Instead, workers should analyze the chasm which exists between their world and the sphere of the press room and consider strategies which bridge this divide. Reporters face many of the same problems as child welfare workers: too little time, deadlines, quick decisions, pressures from above in spite of evidence to the contrary from below. Moreover Aldridge (1990) has observed that social workers do not describe their efforts in clear language and social work itself is not a sufficiently important item for reporters to become expert in its workings. Thus it is dealt with by non-specialist reporters using old clippings for back-ground. Indeed in this case, reporters did not attend the inquiry consistently and stories filed by one reporter were picked up on the Canadian Press news and given far more prominence than their coverage in *The Vancouver Sun*. However, in spite of these challenges, one social worker invited a reporter from the two Vancouver papers, *The Vancouver Sun* and *The Province* to follow him in the course of his duties for a week. Although only *The Province* accepted the offer, the articles written afterwards were largely sympathetic to the challenges facing child welfare workers. This worker attempted to form a relationship with a reporter, not simply plug her with more, seemingly self-serving facts. He invited her into his world. In turn, he may feel more familiar with her struggles and more aware of aspects of his work which make news.

The local neighbourhood press may be more receptive to our overtures as it is always starved for news and less willing to condemn because we, or our families or co-workers, are known locally. Here we are more likely to find ways to keep the press interested in child welfare. As the transcripts revealed, there are many good stories to be told, many bureaucratic impossibilities to expose and many people willing to discuss their frustrations.

Notes

1. We will compare our findings with other studies which analyzed press coverage of child welfare (Franklin and Parton 1991).
2. Except for sources of information, the content analysis is not discussed.
3. After the sentencing of the mother and before the inquiry began, *The Vancouver Sun* set out the victims and villains clearly in an editorial:

> Through the quick wit and wisdom of provincial court judge, Jack McGivern, the killer of a five year old boy has been jailed for ten years. The question is: What will happen to her accomplices?
> Verna Vaudreuil was an obvious villain. Members of her own family reported her for child abuse and tried to take her son away from her.... Yet nothing was done.
> Matthew Vaudreuil spent most of his short life undernourished and bruised from head to toe. That he lived to see his fifth birthday is something of a miracle. That he died at the hands of his mother—after authorities had so many chances to intervene—is a crime.
> What we don't know is how Matthew Vaudreuil slipped through the cracks and, although Social Services Minister Joy MacPhail has ordered an investigation, it is being conducted by members of the same department in which the negligence, if any, occurred. Like the police investigating their own for corruption or brutality, we are inviting the accused to stand as judge and jury. (May 3, 1994: A14)

Headlines in the *The Vancouver Sun* during this period reinforce the messages of the editorial:

ASPHYXIATION: He was hungry, dirty, nervous, then dead. Saturday, April 23, 1994: A2

MATTHEW'S STORY: The boy who was doomed from the start. Saturday, April 30, 1994, Front page, A1

CHILD ABUSE: Police had to make 'deal with the devil.' Monday, May 2, 1994, Front page, B1

MATTHEW VAUDREUIL: Abuse-death report to be censored, MacPhail says. Thursday, May 5, 1994, B5

SOCIAL SERVICES: Improved support for children pledged after boy's death. Friday, May 6, 1994, B2

MATTHEW VAUDREUIL CASE: Ombudsman to probe tortured tot's death: McCallum calls for impartial review, sidesteps minister. Tuesday, May 10, 1994, Front page, A1

MATTHEW VAUDREUIL: Boy's death preventable, father says. Saturday, May 14, 1994, A7

MATTHEW VAUDREUIL: Public inquiry to probe why system failed to save life of abused child. Wednesday, May 18, 1994, B2

Least Disruptive and Intrusive Course of Action . . . for Whom? Insights from Feminist Analysis of Practice in Cases of Child Sexual Abuse

JULIA ELISSA KRANE[1]

Introduction

Across North America, the focus of current child welfare practice reflects a number of dramatic shifts. Broadly speaking, child welfare services have moved from concern for the social welfare of children to a preoccupation with investigating allegations of abuse and neglect, assessing risk to children and providing involuntary protection services instead of voluntary services and resources for families to care for their children (Callahan 1993a; David 1991; Hutchison 1992; Parton and Parton 1988/89). Contemporary "child welfare services are facing spiralling reports of suspected child abuse and neglect with increasingly limited resources" (Trocmé, Tam and McPhee 1995:20). Thus, child welfare agencies are compelled to allocate considerable energy to investigate allegations of abuse and neglect, which results in limiting the funds available for the provision of supportive and protective services (Kammerman and Kahn 1990). Alongside an increase in reports and investigative activities is a transformation in the philosophy, principles and practice around the means to procure the best interests and protection of children. As "evidence has grown of the risks involved in separating children from their families and communities," the maintenance of children with their families has replaced "rescue" as the intervention/philosophy of choice (Jackson 1995:324).

According to Rivers (1993), support of children in their own homes is the most striking change in child welfare work. A topography of clients served by the Children's Aid Society of Metropolitan Toronto, the largest board-operated child welfare agency in North America, reveals that the overwhelming majority are assisted in their own homes (Rivers 1993). During 1992, for example, the agency "worked with close to 20,000 children at risk. Of those, 17,300 were supported in their own families in the community, most of them (83%) living at or below the poverty line. . . . For every child admitted to the care of the state, seven more were maintained in their own family" (Rivers 1993:79).

This ratio is by no means accidental, nor is it confined to a particular child welfare agency as confirmed by similar trends across Canada and the U.K. (Armitage 1993b; Pascall 1986). Aimed at reducing the number of children removed from their families, child welfare statutes direct this shift in practice largely through such notions as family autonomy, least intrusion, permanency for children and family support (Barnhorst and Walter 1991; Rivers 1993). It is a feminist critical analysis of the translation of these principles, in relation to protection practices in cases of child sexual abuse, that forms the crux of this chapter.

A feminist analysis of child welfare practice is one that "places the experience of women, the major group of consumers and providers in the system, at the centre of the inquiry rather than on the fringes" (Callahan 1993b:174). My central thesis is threefold. One, contrary to official child welfare discourse that presents the protection of children as a "public" mandate, protection is actually shifted to and performed by women in the "private" sphere of the family. Two, contrary to official child welfare discourse that presents protection as gender free, the shift in the protection mandate to women as mothers is gendered and engendering: it is very much about women as mothers and the reproduction of women as mothers. Finally, I will suggest that protection efforts which conform to least intrusion and support for children in their homes come about through the obligatory, yet invisible, labour of women in families. These efforts represent practices that are rife with costs and consequences for both women and children.

The chapter begins with a discussion of state/family relations within the context of child welfare practice, followed by a presentation of a case study of child protection interventions undertaken in Ontario in response to child sexual abuse. I conclude with a re-examination of the central axioms upon which child welfare practice is based and suggest implications for policy and practice in the areas of child protection and child sexual abuse.

State Intervention, Family Autonomy and Least Disruption: The Image of Separate Spheres

In Canada, the role of the state in children's welfare and protection has developed gradually. It was not until the early years of the twentieth century that the notion of state responsibility for assuring a minimum standard of well-being for all children was established. At that time, private children's aid societies were organized and provincial child protection legislation was enacted across the country (Bala 1991; Ontario Ministry of Comunity and Social Services 1979). In Ontario, the Act for the Prevention of Cruelty to and Better Protection of Children was passed in 1893, thereby granting children's aid societies the legal authority to remove neglected or abused children from their homes and become their guardians (Bala 1991). This legislation was remarkable; it "empowered private organizations to administer a provincial statute" (Melichercik 1978:190) and crystallized the authorization of state intervention into families in the name of child protection.

Within the last forty years, enormous developments in the field of child protection have occurred (Bala 1991). Extended definitions of abuse and neglect, limitations on temporary care by the state, establishment of criteria for the provision of child protection services via standardized accountability mechanisms, mandatory reporting laws and the development of child abuse registers to track abusers and victims are just some of the changes undertaken in the 1950s and 1960s (Bala 1991; Melichercik 1978; Trocmé 1991).

By the 1970s, attention shifted to the questionable adequacy of the state's child protection efforts that removed children from their families. According to Trocmé (1991), the belief that the state was able to know and provide what was best for children came under close examination and heavy criticism during this decade. As a result, the child welfare system again underwent legal and administrative reforms. In Ontario, key changes included the following: a re-examination of the balance between children's best interests and the least restrictive course of state action; specification of the definition of a child in need of protection; and introduction of the principle of due process (Trocmé 1991).

Together with promotion of "the best interests, protection and well-being of children" and pursuit of "the least restrictive or disruptive course of action," the legislation adopted the following principles: recognition that "while parents often need help in caring for their children, that help should give support to the autonomy and integrity of the family unit and, wherever possible, be provided on the basis of mutual consent"; and "children's services should be provided in a manner that . . . respects children's needs for continuity of care and for stable family relationships" (Ontario 1984:3-4).

Alongside revised principles were modifications to the terms and conditions justifying involuntary intervention in the family. The definition of a child in need of protection was articulated with "more precise and objective" language. This modification aimed to:

> limit intervention to cases in which there is specific harm, or risk of harm, to the child. . . . [It] attempts to limit the range of discretion afforded to judges and social workers, and restricts intervention in the family to relatively well-defined situations. . . . [It] is also consistent with the notion of due process, since it gives parents a clearer idea of the problems they have to address. (Barnhorst and Walter 1991:20)

Apparent through much child welfare discourse is a preoccupation with ascertaining and clarifying the extent of and the limits to state intervention or interference in families and determining the conditions that justify state intervention in family life, the procedures for those interventions and their effects. This emphasis points to the residual nature of child welfare in that meeting children's basic needs and providing for their daily care are responsibilities of parents in the private sphere of the family. Social institutions "only come into play when the normal structures of supply, the family and the market, break down" (Wilensky and Lebeaux 1965:138 cited in Armitage 1993b:42). Thus, the state is authorized to investigate, intervene, protect and provide care only when or after parental care has fallen below a certain standard (Bala 1991; David 1991; Wald 1982).

Though this residual formulation has been remarkably consistent over time and across Canada (Herringer, noted in Wharf 1995), there have been voices of opposition to it.[2] Wharf points out that the residual approach, "anchored in the principle of least intrusiveness," is most paradoxical (1995:5). By refraining from intervening until maltreatment of children has occurred, residual legislation "virtually ensures that intervention will be intrusive" (Wharf 1995:5).

The prevailing assumption of the relationship between state and family is one of separate spheres. Not only are the boundaries between state and family drawn, but their bifurcation is fortified through the principles by which state intervention into the family proceeds—"least disruption," recognition of the family as an independent, self-determining unit, and preferably on the basis of mutual consent. This reification tends to be blind to variations within and between families in terms of gender, socioeconomic status, race, composition and the like. This of course is central when one considers the landscape of the welfare state, particularly the child welfare arm of the state.

Women comprise the majority of unpaid carers, consumers and workers of the social welfare state. "At least 70 percent" of front line child welfare workers in Canada are women (Callahan 1993b:172). The majority of child welfare clients are poor, marginalized, single parent women. Regardless, child welfare analysts have tended to disregard the gendered nature of child welfare and assume that mothers' and children's needs are either synonymous (Hutchison 1992) or that children's needs are best met by their families, particularly their mothers (Contratto 1986; Mandell 1988).

Given that the arena of child welfare is very much a feminized one, analyses of the residual formulation—anchored in the principles of least intrusion and support to help autonomous families—must be considered from the perspectives of women in child welfare. To do otherwise is to maintain the invisibility of women and thus suffer from what Margrit Eichler (1988a) calls gender insensitivity. The research study reported here responds to the legacy of gender invisibility and insensitivity in women's world of child welfare. I ask from the perspectives of women in child welfare, how does the state protect children from sexual abuse? Beyond description, I want to know what social relations are reflected in and reproduced by the procurement of protection in this way.

Re-writing the Problem to Feature Women as Inadequate Wives and Mothers

One of the most profound child welfare problems garnering attention in recent years is the sexual abuse of children and youths. In Canada, the U.S. and the

U.K., we have witnessed a proliferation of inquiries into the extent and nature of child sexual abuse, its consequences and its treatment. Clinicians and researchers have had a great deal to say *about* mothers of sexually abused children (see Krane and Davies 1995 for a discussion of this discourse). However, it is not until very recently that investigations, largely undertaken by feminists, have produced accounts *from* mothers of sexually abused children.[3] The analysis presented here contributes to this developing knowledge base.[4]

Protection, as I will illustrate below, is a process that entails translation of the problem of *child sexual abuse* to one of *failure to protect*. Rewritten in this way, the problem is transformed from an offence committed predominantly by men to transgressions or acts of omission by women as wives, mothers and protectors. It is thus no wonder that the ensuing intervention scrutinizes and maintains women as mother protectors.

Since the mid-1960s, spurred on by child protectionists and women's advocates, understandings of the problem of child sexual abuse have shifted. Once considered rare, child sexual abuse is now recognized as a complex psychosocial and legal problem that reflects the organization of male sexuality, vulnerability of children and impoverished or threatening personal relations (Finkelhor 1984; Glaser and Frosh 1993).

Numerous explanations are in circulation at this time. Though not mutually exclusive, they may be categorized according to a primary emphasis on offender characteristics (intrapsychic and physiological), and on his interpersonal and familial relationships (family dynamics). In the child welfare context, the family dynamics analysis is the prevalent model used to explain child sexual abuse. According to MacLeod and Saraga (1988), this framework has achieved the status of common sense in both lay and professional discourse. It prevails in training materials for child welfare practitioners (Krane 1994).

In this analysis, the family as a social unit is considered dysfunctional: fathers are described as dominant and controlling or dependent and weak; mothers as unavailable and helpless or powerful and overbearing; and daughters as vulnerable. All family members are thought to perpetuate the abuse for fear of family breakup. While it is beyond the scope of this chapter to detail the family systems analysis and the many criticisms that have been levelled against it,[5] it is important to point out that sexual abuses perpetrated by father or father figures account for about only one-tenth to one-quarter of sexual offences committed against children (see Krane 1994 for a more thorough examination of this issue). In considering alternative analyses and practices at the conclusion of this chapter, I shall revisit this issue.

As with the dominant discourse in the field, the child protection workers who participated in the study on which this analysis is based typically described their cases in terms of family dynamics and dysfunction: "These are usually very dysfunctional families. The sexual abuse is a symptom of a much larger problem in the family, problems mostly between the mother and the father, and the father as an individual"; or, "I don't just get the facts, I look at the family dynamics that contribute to the abuse." In expanding on the features of the dysfunctional family, workers made reference to what Glaser and Frosh (1993) call "microsocial factors," where the focus is on the functioning of individual protagonists (especially the abuser) and their interpersonal relationships. In doing so, women's inadequacies as wives and mothers are worked into the problem. Witness the following accounts by workers of their cases:

> They had a very unstable relationship, actually violent. He was very controlling and he met his needs through the kids. . . . Maybe because of the dysfunctional relationship with [his wife], it was easier to look to his children.

> The father was overpowering and powerful and to a large extent this caused the abuse. In fact, he conditioned [his daughter] from an early age to accept nudity, and that's what I mean by "abuse of power" but you see, [the mother] never said anything except "I think you should put on some clothes" and that's all she did.

This last excerpt refers to a case of sexual abuse perpetrated by a stepfather on his teenaged stepdaughter. During the investigation, the worker recalled how the teenager "trembled with fear." Having witnessed the abuse of her mother, she was afraid of her stepfather's "violent temper" and worried about the consequences of disclosure. When the worker first met the stepfather, an alleged wife batterer and child sexual abuser, she was "taken aback": "I expected this monstrous and frightening man to walk into my office. Instead, what I got was a pipsqueak! Skinny and scruffy! [His wife] could floor him if she really wanted to!" Seen in the above cited passage is a shift in focus from offender to non-offender; it comes about through dissatisfaction with a mother who failed to stand up to or control her husband, i.e., mother "never said anything except . . . and that's all she did" or she "could floor him if she really wanted to." That he reportedly victimized her is overlooked *and* she is seen as not having done enough to put a stop to the abuse.

To confront and regulate an abuser is to assume that women are vested with great powers, another one of which is clairvoyance:

> [The mother] left her husband alone with the child on a regular basis and he encouraged her to do that. He gave her money to go out and play bingo and it was too good to be true. He gave her money to go out and play bingo! Well, did she not stop to ask what's going on? (Intake worker)

A shift in focus from the actions and responsibilities of the offender as a man, father and husband to the non-offending woman's failure as mother and wife is again revealed. *She* left her child with the husband; *she* failed to question his motives. While it is not so incredible that a husband might encourage a wife to enjoy herself, it is remarkable that the mother becomes responsible for the abuse for having failed to question or police her husband and hence protect the child.

To expect women to be all-knowing and all-powerful flies in the face of the dynamics of child sexual abuse wherein the offender sets up the conditions for access, opportunity and privacy, induces or engages the child and imposes secrecy (Sgroi, Blick and Porter 1985). It also denies the complexities of women's experiences following children's disclosures of child sexual abuse. As documented elsewhere, women's awareness of and reactions to child sexual abuse vary (Carter 1990; Faller 1988; Hooper 1992; Jacobs 1990; Johnson 1992; Krane 1994; Myer 1985). Yet, regardless of the dynamics of abuse and variations in the mother's knowledge of abuse, the expectation that the mother knew, should have known or should have detected "warning signs" was thematic. Workers commented: "Despite their denial, many mothers have had the warning signs" or "I wonder did she have any sense about what was going on? Weren't there any warning signs or red flags?" For mothers, the effect was one of blame, as seen in the following passages from two of the mothers interviewed:

> [The worker] asked "do you know what's happening to your daugh-ter?" I said no, but she was just like a drill soldier, coming after me, and she said "you have to know what happened to your daughter". . . . She yelled at me and accused me of knowing. She was very forceful. I got angry and asked her "why are you blaming me?"

> They automatically assumed that I am to blame, that I must have known. That's how they see it and it really bothered me.

The expectation of the mother to identify signs of abuse denies the likelihood that such signs are indicators of abuse either to the highly trained eye or after the fact. Even skilled professionals know this. As one caseworker recalled, "I was working with the family and I knew [the boy] had problems controlling his bowels. This is a real clue to sexual abuse and I never figured it out . . . I should have picked up the clues, I should have known."

A surface view analysis illustrates that women are worked into the problem, their inadequacies are featured, they are expected to have known and acted accordingly by questioning the husband's behaviour or altering their own. Thus, the problem of child sexual abuse is being rewritten in a way that women become responsible for the abuse and its resolution. Beneath the surface, a particular form of gender relations is operative. Women are viewed almost exclusively as (defective) mothers and wives. Featuring women's inadequacies is very much in harmony with pervasive cultural attitudes about women as mothers in contemporary Western societies. These include the idealization and glorification of mothering and the invisibility of mothering labour (Krane and Davies 1995). It is no wonder that, despite shifts in understanding the sexual abuse of children, women continue to be implicated in a problem of male perpetrated sexual offences against children. This paradigm reflects a legacy of normative and decontextualized expectations of women as "good mothers." Mothering, including the care and protection of children, does not occur in a vacuum. As Humphreys suggests, "the gap between these expectations and the status, power, personal and material resources to fulfil them yawns like a chasm for many women" (1994:53). Social workers are no exception. Given our own internalized normative expectations of mothers, any woman's failure to recognize signs of abuse is frustrating and disappointing, yet beyond question. Embroiling mothers so centrally into the problem of child sexual abuse is far from a neutral activity. It reinforces and reproduces women's responsibilities as mothers for the well-being of the family in the private sphere.

Intervention: Transferring the Protection Mandate

To protect children from sexual abuse is ostensibly to bring about an end to the maltreatment in the least harmful manner. The immediate protection of the child is accomplished, according to investigation and intervention protocols, by separating the victim and the offender and providing support for the non-offending parent. This route to protection conforms to least intrusion, support for children in their own homes and continuity of care.

An examination of how protection actually comes about reveals that it falls largely on the shoulders of women. Women are transformed into mother protectors, a process that is comprised of a nexus of interrelated features: establishing the protection priority for mother; bypassing any meaningful exploration of her reactions and needs; eliciting expressions of belief and support for the child from the mother; and requiring mothers to protect versus presenting women with a "choice" between the child and the offender. As I will suggest, the gendered and engendering nature of protection is far from being least intrusive and supportive for women.

Throughout their case discussions, for example, workers spoke of the central importance of mothers in securing the child's safety in the least intrusive manner for children:

> I ask: Do I see any strengths in mom? Is she an ally? Am I going to get her on side for this kid? She is crucial, mother is crucial.... If you don't have her on side, you might as well take that kid out.

> The mandate says we have to make child protection decisions right away, and if that mother can't protect, we don't leave the kid there.

Mom may need some time, but right now, we're under pressure to protect children.

Under pressure to protect, the worker is faced with evaluating, enlisting and transforming mother as protector. This process is discernable in an interview with a senior intake worker:

Oh, the father has to leave. If he won't leave, she [the mother] has to leave [with the children]. You just don't leave the kid in the same house [as the offender]. The key figure is the mother, of course. . . . You must get her on side . . . .

I tell the mother that we believe the daughter . . . [is] telling the truth, and it's extremely important that you, of all people, believe her. You may have some ambivalent feelings, but you need to put those aside, we'll work on that later. . . . [You must] tell her you love her and you believe her. . . . If the wrong response comes out, wow, we're in trouble!

A number of key features of protection become visible here. The centrality of the mother to the protection process is undeniable, as is apparent the pressure on the mother to protect. At the same time, her experience is disregarded, i.e., "we'll work on that later." This theme of dependence upon and disregard for the mother is pervasive:

The child and her protection are my first and foremost concerns. We say "look lady, you're responsible for protecting your child. . . ." Our job is to get her to say all the right things, we'll deal with her issues later.

We say we support moms, but what we really say is "you need to be here for your child." Even if she is reeling from the disclosure, we want her to focus on her child. The expectation in the first several hours is for mother to go through all these emotions and come out the other end saying "I believe my child!"

Several contradictions are apparent. The very urgent, critical and fast paced nature of child protection investigations preclude any substantial evaluation of the mother's protective stance. Yet this evaluation figures prominently in deciding the immediate plan of action for the child (see Cage 1988; Everson et al. 1989; Horejsi et al. 1987; Pellegrin and Wagner 1990). As well, this evaluation is undertaken at a time of crisis when the mother is most vulnerable, least informed and not necessarily equipped with the means to protect (Krane 1990, 1994). Finally, the mother is needed to protect (to support and believe the child and effect a separation from the offender) while attention to her predicament, with its attending casualties, falls by the wayside.

Another feature of the protection process is that of the obligatory versus voluntary acceptance of the protection mandate. Though workers spoke of giving mothers a choice, interventions more aptly reflected coercion or an unquestioned expectation to protect, as is evident in the following passages from interviews with the social workers:

> I think we tend to expect a lot from the mothers because they're mothers and they're supposed to protect and that's their role in life.

> I didn't even have to threaten her [the mother] with apprehension of the children.

> We put her in the position of feeling judged that she is not a caring and good mother if she chooses this adult man over this helpless child.

For mothers, choice was mere rhetoric. The following statements from mothers show that the message to protect the victim by separating from the offender is clear, intense and potent: "They gave me an ultimatum: either my husband had to leave the house or my daughter had to leave," or "When CAS [the Children's Aid Society] found out, they wanted him out . . . and you got no say."

The expectation for the mother to support the child and separate from her partner was accompanied by an assumption that mother protection entails minimal disruption and requires minimal aid. On the first theme, these were some of the caseworkers' impressions: "I think she was relieved that it all came out"; "It didn't affect her one bit"; "I'd say there was no reaction." Rarely was this the case from the perspectives of the mothers themselves. Described as "hell" or "the floor caved in on me," women were faced with loss of their home or job or husband or children. Some moved into public housing, others sought welfare. Some had to contend with finding accommodation, paying first and last month's rent, packing belongings and physically relocating while working full-time or caring for their children. Throughout this period they also had to attend support groups to deal with the abuse, arrange for their children to attend group meetings and appear in court.

Mothers reported that help in obtaining welfare, housing, daycare and transportation for regular and mandatory meetings at the agency was not available. The dearth of help was overwhelming, as conveyed in the following statements: "as far as I'm concerned, the agency did nothing. They just told me to move out"; "I got nothing from them, well, not true, I got the shaft."

Women spoke of how their lives were dramatically altered as a result of assuming this protection mandate. There was the loss of paid employment, loss of freedom (i.e., "I'm stuck right back being at home"), loneliness and despair in the destruction of their families as they knew them, and the loss of the right to determine what was in the best interests of themselves, their children and partners. They also noted adjustments to their daily routines that were necessary to fulfil the protection mandate. Accommodation of protection is apparent as one mother discusses how she protects her stepdaughters from her son (the offender):

> I'm the one who always protects them. I arrange for the babysitter. I worry about getting home on time.... [My husband] says five minutes won't matter, but I say it does. This is a big change for me in my life.

> I've had to give up [my weekend job] because if [my husband] has to go out on the weekends with the Boy Scouts, camping or something, he doesn't ask "are you going to be home?" He just expects me to be there. I know better than to plan things for myself because I have to watch the kids.

In sum, she described the mandate to be like a "ball and chain," confining her to the home to watch, police and protect. Protection as women's work, obligation and responsibility is a recurrent theme. It is apparent in the mothers' pledges of allegiance to protect:

> I know the warning signs now; if he starts drinking or smoking [pot] again or if he's depressed . . . if anything like this happens, I'm supposed to talk to him and call the agency. I'm supposed to look out for him and how he's feeling.

> I wouldn't go out anywhere and if I did go out, I'd do it when they're at school and I'd be home in time for their lunch or I'd take them with me.

That women pledge to remain at home and keep a watchful eye on all members—clearly unrealistic—reflects the internalization of the expectation to protect and the potency of state interventions that transform mothers into protectors.

The strategy of transforming women into mother protectors was not without criticism from social workers. One worker recognized how mothers are "overlooked" during the investigation. Another worker acknowledged that mothers are in a "no win situation of having to choose between their husbands and their children." She elaborated as follows:

> A woman has operated all her life a certain way, she may be subservient, and to ask her overnight to stand on her own two feet is devastating. She needs a lot of support and we use coercion . . . .

> I've learned . . . that this is difficult for everyone. . . . Mothers are put
> through so much more than the alleged offender and I want to deal with
> her feelings but I push past them because there are concerns about the
> risk and protection of the child.

Despite recognition that the circumstances facing mothers are particularly difficult, hesitation, vacillation and failure by the mother to protect were identified as the most troublesome aspects of the job by workers. For mothers, the dearth of help associated with the swift separation of child and offender, together with feeling disregarded, blamed and fearful of losing their children, worked as deterrents for talking with and confiding in their workers.

Mothers' experiences of blame and failure coupled with workers' disappointment and frustration drive a harmful and costly wedge between the two. Ironically, this wedge alienates mothers in a protection process that rests with them.

Re-examining Separate Spheres: Women and the Child Welfare State

A key issue that emerges in child welfare discourse is the place of the state in the private lives of families. Child welfare analysts deliberate the definitions of mistreatment, situations that justify state intervention and the principles upon which such interventions should proceed. A perusal of child welfare discourse reveals repeated references to state "intrusion," "coercion" and "disruption." As well, analysts ponder the benefit-to-harm ratio of state interventions into families and the relative merits of an interventionist versus non-interventionist/ family autonomy approach to definitions of a child in need of protection.

In this discourse, state intrusion—from more or less coercion or disruption— has been constructed as if it is separable from the autonomous and private family. While the state is not supposed to infiltrate the privacy of the family or familial responsibility for the care of children, the statutory mandate to investigate, assess and intervene in order to protect children supersedes the "privacy" of the family. The protection mandate underscores and legitimizes the state's manipulation of the boundary between public and private spheres.

When we talk of intrusion and coercion, disruption and restriction, benefits and risks, a non-interventionist state and family autonomy, we must ask "from whose perspective are these distinctions drawn"? These debates seem to have been argued without concern for the primary caretakers of children—women and mothers. As traced in this study, the protection mandate is transferred to women in families. The shift tells us a great deal about broader social relations, in particular the workings of the welfare state vis-à-vis women.

First, child welfare practices that give rise to protection through the mother are by no means neutral or haphazard. Rather, they are *dependent* upon mothers for successful protection of children. Dependence upon the mother for protection, coupled with an assumption that she is ready, willing and able to devote herself wholly to this task, is consistent with traditional assumptions of women's role in the family. Women are seen to be primarily responsible for and most capable of tending to physical, emotional and other needs of the young, the infirm and the aged. These assumptions coexist with everyday practices in cases of child sexual abuse that reinforce children's need for continuous care by their mothers and the availability of mothers to provide such care and protection. To understand that protection is actually accomplished through women in families is to appreciate that the state depends on women to protect, in the name of that which is best for children. Everyday child protection practices, even in progressive practice settings, reproduce a gendered division of labour wherein women are relegated to and held responsible for the family.

Second, further empirical support of feminist critiques of the problematic bifurcation of public/state and private/family is provided by the fact that it is women who are placed in the protector role. This role underlines the complexity of women's relationship to the welfare state as unpaid carers, consumers and intermediaries or patchworkers. From the identification and accentuation of the problem of child sexual abuse in terms of the mother's failure to protect, to interventions aimed at enlisting her protection, it is assumed that she is the best, if not the only, appropriate protector for the child. It is assumed that regardless of her relationship to the public sphere in general, and wage labour in particular, she can and will bridge the (state) mandate to protect with the need of the child for protection. This is no small matter given that most women with children work outside the home (Eichler 1988b).

Transformation of the mother into a protector unravels the division between the public and private spheres. This process calls into question the essence of a "state service" as distinct from women's servicework, exposing core assumptions that underlie welfare state policies such as protection. As *it is the mother who provides the fundamental service* (albeit an unpaid and invisible one), contemporary debates about the nature and extent of state intervention in families and conceptions of an interventionist state (as relieving or supporting the family) make little sense. The notion of "least intrusive" belies women's experiences of protection and the labour associated with it. Feminist analysts have long pointed to the fact that "support for the family" is really support for family responsibility, and support for family responsibility is really women's responsibility as wives, daughters or mothers to care for children, the aged or the ill (Baines, Evans and Neysmith 1991; Pascall 1986). "Mother" is always expected to remain "in character" and is not expected "to need or have the right to need social services or social funds" (Rosenberg 1988:387). Sassoon (1987) goes so far as to suggest that it is only in the absence of women in families that the state will provide fundamental services and funds.

That the state depends on mothers to protect suggests that "the domestic sphere, the world of work, the welfare state are all organized as if women were continuing a traditional role" (Sassoon 1987:160) as full-time mothers and housewives. The impression given is that women's participation in the paid labour force is marginal, and that they are ready, willing and able to relinquish paid work and depend upon a male wage in order to make themselves available to protect. Clearly, then, the gendered and engendering subtext of the welfare state plays a large part in sustaining "the dependent position of women within the family" (Pascall 1986:28).

Assuming that women's relation to the world of paid work is marginal has many implications. There are extensive and often unrecognized personal costs to women. Mother protection entails taking on other domestic-related unpaid labour for the best interests of children, with little regard for that which might be in the mother's own interests.

There are other costs too. It could be argued that the allocation of protection to mothers is a cost saving measure for the state in that expenses related to substitute care are saved. To cease depending on women as unpaid protectors would be costly to the state. However, the state does expend a certain amount of money on the social work labour required to investigate and assess allegations of abuse. Normally this money is allocated to administrative employment and infrastructure costs and is *not designated for the recipients of service*, namely women and their children.

Finally, I would argue that the intervention model of mother protector may actually cost the state. This model assumes women's nonessential labour force participation, requires separation of the child from the offender and results in potential loss of at least one if not the only source of income. In so doing, it renders women and children dependent upon someone or something for income, including the state (i.e., welfare, mother's allowance, subsidized housing and the like). Recognizing that the women who participated in this study were economically disadvantaged, as are many women who come in contact with the child welfare system, the removal of one (or the only) breadwinner must necessarily heighten the costs of the intervention for these women.

Implications for Policy and Practice

The child welfare system is not responsible for changing the prevailing distribution of power that maintains hierarchical and oppressive gender relations, nor does this arm of the state meet "all of the needs of families and children" (Callahan 1993b:203). Nevertheless, it can and must "do its part in making change" (Callahan 1993b:203). Callahan calls for feminists to rethink rather than reject child welfare services. In this spirit, I conclude with a discussion of the implications of this analysis for child protection policy and practice.

With cutbacks in the public sector and changes in funding arrangements between federal and provincial levels of government, not to mention the insidiousness of "family values," state policies can be expected to continue to promote the family "through framing social policies on the assumption that women perform unpaid labour in the home and are economically dependent on men" (Dale and Foster 1986:61). As such, women can expect to take on heavier burdens as carers (Land 1991). While it is arguable that the mother should not be seen as the only or the best protector (Krane 1994), the aforementioned structures and ideologies provide few, if any, alternatives around achieving protection. In closing, I shall consider the needs of mothers as protectors within the context of current practice.

To begin with, it is imperative to explicitly identify the mother as protector in order to view her relation to the state differently. Women in this context should not be considered simply as "mother," whose needs are either assumed to be analogous to her child's (eclipsed by those of her child) or disregarded. Rather they should be understood as a *state resource* or *central feature of the intervention model* to protect. This designation entails revealing rather than concealing the transfer of the protection mandate. Adding women to the equation of protection thus produces the opportunity to contemplate and better provide for mothers in order for them to fulfil the protection mandate. It also thwarts the all too easy dismissal of the costs and consequences for women of accepting the protection mandate.

Recording what women need, along with the costs and consequences to them, is markedly different from practice that posits protection as state responsibility and state intervention as relief for the family. In no way do the transfer and allocation of protection to women entail relief, regardless of how manageable protection might be for them. Rather, protection is plainly added onto women's workloads and must be regarded as an additional feature of women's labour. This is difficult, for it requires a shift in conceptualizing women's expected caring and servicing; mother protection is not invisible nor performed out of "love and self-denial and care for the needs of others" but it is "work" (Balbo 1987:52).

Though women's needs regarding income, housing, daycare, transportation etc. will vary to a certain extent, it does not seem to be in the interests of women and children to assign mothers this mandate without tangible aid. Child welfare most often deals with the results of poverty and marginalization (Wharf 1995). This impoverishment is often heightened because successful protection typically entails immediate separation of the child from the offender (an offender who may have been a breadwinner), and the separation tends to be an extended one. Consequently, addressing the material conditions of mother protecting is necessary. A few suggestions include developing housing policies that give preference to emergency situations, the establishment of safe shelters for women with sexually abused children, routine requests for court ordered support payments for mother protectors and alternative and non-stigmatizing care plans.

Exposing the gendered and engendering process of transforming women into mother protectors is to compel us to re-orient our understanding of the problem of child sexual abuse and our responses to it. The roles and responsibilities of fathers (biological, step- or adoptive fathers) must also be factored into the protection equation.

A number of issues arise. Given that the majority of sexual offences against children are male perpetrated, one might wonder how fathers can be considered protectors of children. However, because fathers or father figures do not account for the majority of offenders, they can be expected, if not obligated, to engage in the protection process. While protection by parent(s) is preferable to protection by the state, it does not logically flow that the mother is the only protector available in most cases. This means that the non-offending father/figure can be called upon to support and believe his child and participate more fully in protection.

Involving men in the care and protection of children is neither straightforward nor readily accepted among feminists. It does not simply entail sharing burdens and responsibilities in the domestic sphere. Rather, as Eisenstein (1981:187) points out, when we ask men to "help" rear children, we must understand that we are "speaking of a fundamental reorganization of society."

> The entire social organization of the way people live their lives, as well as think about them, is involved. The organization of wage labour, the relationship between home and work, the conception of public life, and the definition of masculine and feminine have to be completely rethought and restructured. (Eisenstein 1981:187)

The equation of "father" with "offender" is a central component of the dominant conceptualization of the problem of child sexual abuse. The configuration of father–daughter incest shapes our understanding of the problem of child sexual abuse, regardless of the various forms of such abuse. Differences between the dynamics and effects of father–daughter incest and those sexual abuses perpetrated by non-parental relatives and non-relatives must be considered when rethinking child protection policy and practice. It is by challenging the predominant image of child sexual abuse as a problem of dysfunctional families, implicating mothers in particular, that we may find ways to construct women as mothers differently. As long as protection is realized through mothers in the private sphere, neither the state nor men will have to carry the costs nor share in the protection of children.

Notes

1. The author gratefully acknowledges Health and Welfare Canada for financial support for this research.
2. The residual approach has been criticized for de-emphasizing the social relations, structural or material factors that shape the well-being and care of children (Callahan 1993b; David 1991; Smith and Smith 1990; Swift 1991; Wharf 1993a)

and for establishing the idea that normal standards of parental care—and instances when these standards have been breached—can be defined (Armitage 1993b; David 1991).

3. See Cammaert 1988; Carter 1990; Faller 1988; Gavey et al. 1990; Hooper 1992; Jacobs 1990; Johnson 1992; Krane 1994; Myer 1985; Wattenberg 1985.

4. This analysis is based on a study conducted at a child welfare agency in rural Ontario. The organization took a leadership role in developing and implementing a coordinated approach to responding to child sexual abuse: its front line staff received ongoing training in the area of child sexual abuse; and a protocol for investigation and intervention was followed, whereby protection of children was secured through the separation of the offender from the victim in order to enable the victim to remain with her/his family.

    Data were collected between 1989-1990. Thirty-nine interviews were conducted with eight mothers of sexually abused children and their female social workers. These interviews invited discussion on the women's thoughts on the problem of child sexual abuse and their experiences as workers and clients in dealing with the problem. As well, workers brought to their discussions two other cases of child sexual abuse that were examined. Of the cases discussed, thirteen male perpetrators were identified: five biological fathers; two stepfathers; one brother; one step-brother; one friend of a brother; one grandfather; one paternal uncle; one cousin. Data from these interviews were analyzed qualitatively and juxtaposed against an analysis of organizational, professional and legislative documents such as case records, court files and training, policy and procedural manuals for protection workers. Adopting a critical case study design, the focus of the research is on tracing the process of protection and explicating the social relations beneath the surface view of protection.

5. For details on the family systems analysis and criticisms of it, see Gavey et al. 1990; Jacobs 1990; Krane 1990; MacLeod and Saraga 1988.

The Gove Report
and First Nations Child Welfare

GLEN SCHMIDT

Introduction

In recent years First Nations in Canada have sought to gain control of child welfare services. These efforts have met with varying degrees of success, but clearly First Nations continue to have a subordinate relationship to provincial governments, particularly in the areas of child welfare legislation and practice standards. For this reason, First Nations people view changes in legislation, practice standards and service delivery methods in child welfare with intense interest and sometimes suspicion, particularly when they are fuelled by majority sentiment and interests and when they run counter to their cultural and value base. The recent Gove Report (1995) into child welfare practice in British Columbia provides these challenges for First Nations.

This report is a sweeping document with the potential to influence major changes in the delivery of child welfare services. First Nations have regarded Gove's recommendations with concern because, although they focus on the Ministry of Social Services, their contents have implications for established and emerging First Nations child welfare agencies throughout British Columbia. Some of the recommendations may run counter to First Nations child welfare practice yet, at the same time, First Nations are prepared to work alongside the province as they attempt to build a more effective response to the needs of their children.

Background on the Gove Report

On May 19, 1994, Minister of Social Services Joy MacPhail responded to media and political pressure by appointing Judge Thomas Gove to head an independent commission of inquiry into the death of five and one-half year old Matthew Vaudreuil. Matthew died on July 9, 1992 as a result of injuries inflicted by his mother Verna Vaudreuil. Gove was instructed to "inquire into, report and make recommendations on the adequacy of services and the policies and practices of the Ministry of Social Services in the area of child protection, as they related to Matthew"(Gove 1995:2). However, the scope of the inquiry expanded and Judge Gove embarked upon a more comprehensive and systemic examination of child welfare practice in British Columbia.

The findings of the report raise serious concerns about child welfare practice. According to the documentation provided to the Gove Commission, Matthew Vaudreuil had contact with twenty-one social workers and twenty-four physicians during his brief life. His mother, who had herself been a child in care, sometimes sought assistance and support in parenting Matthew who engaged in difficult tantrums and self-abusive behaviour. Verna Vaudreuil faced serious obstacles as a parent, given her own life circumstances. She experienced physical and sexual abuse as a child and later as an adult. She was mentally challenged and lacked many basic life skills including the ability to adequately parent Matthew. Retrospectively, it appears that obvious concerns like Matthew's failure to thrive, his frustrating behaviour, malnutrition, neglect and Verna's poor understanding of normative child development and needs were observed and documented. However, Matthew remained with his mother who continued to receive a variety of services that were poorly coordinated, lacked a mechanism for communicating critical information and failed to produce lasting or beneficial change.

In his conclusions Judge Gove blames a system that had lost sight of why a child protection service exists. He contends that the system, the minister and the workers offered services that were not child-centred but were directed primarily to achieve benefit for Matthew's mother. Gove believes that this type of environment resulted in a situation where Matthew's well-being became secondary to the parent's and, consequently, the young boy lost his life. His criticisms are not constructed from the perspective of parental pathology so much as they are based on serving the interests and needs of the child ahead of those of the parent.

In Canada provincial governments have launched numerous reviews[1] of child welfare practice, most resulting from tragedies similar to Matthew's or a series of questionable practices that collectively raise public concern about the child welfare system. To a large extent the Gove Inquiry into Child Protection does not represent anything new. However, Gove's work is thorough in the area of statutory child protection and the 118 recommendations that flow from the document are directed toward establishing higher standards of quality assurance in the delivery of child protection services. The organization of the ministry, communication methods, the training of social workers, police and medical personnel, strengthened child advocacy and professional regulation are some of the highlights that emerge from Gove. Overall the report tends to confine itself to protection services and seldom ventures into the broader domain of child welfare. Issues related to the current malaise of the Canadian social welfare system such as child poverty and access to affordable daycare receive scant mention. Throughout the document one is often left with the impression that child protection is somehow an entity unto itself, separate and divorced from other elements of social policy that affect the lives of children. In fairness to Judge Gove, he was not called upon to develop a global assessment of the state of children in British Columbia but, within the context of such reviews, there certainly is latitude to pursue a more complete examination.

Children's Rights

On one level, Gove, and reports of a similar nature, advocate strongly for children's as opposed to parental rights. Young people like Matthew are seen to be without a voice and therefore struggle within a context of heightened vulnerability. The view that children have rights is a relatively recent development that requires profound changes in attitude and policy before it can be fully realized. However, this particular view of children's rights represents a position that is eurocentric. This in itself is not wrong and certainly should not lead one to condemn Gove's conclusions. However, the view of children and child protection put forward in the Gove Report and others like it must be placed in a context where practice can be considered from the perspective of alternative historical and cultural points of view. Not all cultures or peoples have developed from the same roots.

Historically, European practices of childrearing have regarded children as chattels whose wills needed to be controlled and moulded to meet the needs of parents, authority figures and the prevailing social order (Radbill 1987; Miller 1984). The Judeo Christian tradition was used to support the development of patriarchal family structures in which the father had supreme control and could dominate his wife and children through threat and violence. By extension, all parents, including those who are sole parents, have authority over their children and as a society we have tended to perpetuate a view of children as family property. Gove challenges these traditional views (at least as they relate to the parent–child relationship), and suggests that parental rights have been awarded precedence over the rights of children who are powerless to speak for themselves. This view is elaborated in his criticism of various child welfare practice models used by the ministry in British Columbia. The "strengths" and "brokerage" models of case management, as well as the "family group conference" model, are seen as symptoms of a system that neglects the fundamental rights of children. The premise is that, in supporting the parents, the family and by extension the health and well-being of children is strengthened. Many aspects of this approach are compatible with other cultural views of child welfare, particularly those of First Nations who regard the larger community as parent. Given this reality, one is left with the problem of determining how Gove fits with the First Nations view of child welfare practice.

First Nations Child Welfare

There is no single model of First Nations child welfare that can be held up as the paradigm for practice. This should not be surprising as First Nations are not a homogenous group but represent a variety and range of cultures and historical experiences. Though one cannot point to a single, clear model of First Nations child welfare practice, there is an abundance of critical analysis documenting the abuses experienced by First Nations families and children. Policy makers have been told what First Nations do not want to see in terms of child welfare services. This body of literature has tended to be largely analytic and highly critical of historic service provision, political relationships and child maltreatment (Timpson 1995). Child welfare services in particular have been seen as an extension of colonialism, and as a way to incorporate First Nations into the social and economic system of the dominant culture (Hudson and McKenzie 1981).

Together with the residential school system, child welfare practices promoted assimilation and cultural genocide. Patrick Johnston (1983) used the term "sixties scoop" to describe the disproportionate number of First Nations children who were brought into care by child welfare agencies. Many of these children were adopted outside of their culture, and in some provinces, like Manitoba, they were shipped right out of the country. In 1982 the strong objections of First Nations to such practices led to the Kimelman review and the subsequent report, *No Quiet Place* (1985), which called for the immediate cessation of out of province adoptions. Other abuses of First Nation's children within the child welfare system gained considerable exposure and media attention with the death of children like Richard Cardinal. His death represented a failure of the system and resulted in yet another provincial review of child welfare practice.

During the 1980s the media portrayal of tragedies such as Richard Cardinal's death, combined with the will and determination of First Nations to control and deliver child welfare services, led to the development of First Nations child welfare agencies and the possibility that alternative models of practice would emerge. A number of authors describe the different arrangements relating to jurisdiction and mandate that have evolved with the transfer and devolution of child welfare service to First Nations (Durst, McDonald and Rich 1995; Wharf 1989. Hudson and Taylor-Henley (1987a) suggest that models of control can be grouped under three broad categories: "autonomous"; "delegated authority"; and "integrated." The autonomous model is a truly independent model subject only to law and authority arising out of self-governing First Nations. As this model does not exist in practice, First Nations child welfare has been subject to the same principles as child welfare administered within the provincial jurisdiction. The operative models are those of delegated authority and integration. The model of delegated authority authorizes First Nations child welfare agencies to implement and administer child welfare service on behalf of the provincial government. An integrated model uses the existing structure with the addition of indigenous case aides, advisory committees and elders to work alongside the provincial worker in a support capacity. These circumstances have largely compelled First Nations child welfare agencies to operate according to provincial legislation, standards and practices. Hudson and Taylor-Henley (1995) point to a 1989 Indian and Northern Affairs Canada document which specifically states that a central principle of First Nations child welfare practice is that it will follow provincial legislation.[2]

First Nations child welfare agencies have not been immune to tragedies that result in the type of scrutiny exemplified by the Gove Report. For example, the 1988 suicide of Lester Desjarlais led to an inquiry and a report under the Fatality Inquiries Act (Giesbrecht 1992). Like Gove, Judge Giesbrecht takes a view that places the child at the centre of the child welfare system. In his report he was highly critical of the First Nations child welfare agency, Dakota Ojibway Child and Family Services (DOCFS), and their methods of conducting child welfare practice. He described political interference in case planning and a system that neglected documentation to the detriment of children and their families.

However, Isaac Beaulieu, an official with DOCFS, passed the record keeping criticism off as an example of a cultural value clash between an oral tradition and one based upon the written word. On the other hand, critical responses from members of First Nations demonstrated that there was no unanimity on this issue.[3] Disagreement regarding methods and treatment is also common among non-First Nations people. Yet because First Nations approaches may differ from traditional approaches, they receive closer scrutiny that highlights and some-times calls into question the validity of different views. This is illustrated by differences between First Nations and the dominant culture in the proposed treatment of sexual offenders and their victims. For example, the Canadian justice system model is adversarial and, if found guilty, the offender faces punishment and retribution. The public has increasingly called for longer sentences and publication of identifying information prior to release of offend-ers who have sexually abused children. However, within some First Nations communities the direction has been one of achieving reconciliation and healing (Taylor-Henley and Hill 1990). Approaches to treatment or healing are holistic, community-owned and community-based. Individual pathology is not empha-sized in approaches that use the medicine wheel as a framework for change (Longclaws 1994). Similar models in other First Nations communities have developed through the use of sentencing circles and other holistic community based approaches.

First Nations seem to have a somewhat different view of justice from the dominant culture and this leads to what Associate Chief Judge Murray Sinclair (1989) has described as cultural conflict. Misunderstanding arises around concepts such as non-interference and the role of contemporary legislated services (Ross 1992; Brant 1990). Sinclair (1989), Brant (1990) and Ross (1992) argue that law, the application of law and the resulting services are cultural constructs imposed by the dominant culture. It is the dominant culture that must begin to understand and accept that there are alternative and equally valid ways of achieving justice. At the same time, critical questions can be asked about the fact that, in the case of sexual abuse, offenders are almost entirely male, and whether alternative models afford sufficient protection to women and children. Indeed, First Nations women have asked these types of questions. There are concerns that implementation of alternative methods of justice will serve to support the system of patriarchy that has arisen out of the Indian Act. Sentencing circles, banishment and reconciliation may not be enough to provide reasonable assurance of protection to all women and children.

Despite the fact that there is not one archetypal model of First Nations child welfare, and there are clearly divergent views within First Nations regarding alternative approaches, it is apparent that there are some commonalities that are rooted in important values. A key feature of the common value base relates to the place of children within the community and the family. The report *Liberating Our Children, Liberating Our Nations* (Aboriginal Community Panel 1992:10) describes the relation of children to their culture in this way:

> Traditionally, the care of a child is the overall responsibility of an extended family, with members of that extended family playing various roles. In the event that any member of the family might be disabled or absent, there are many more people to take on their responsibilities. More importantly, it was never necessary to surrender children to the care of strangers. There were always people to whom the child was bonded and amongst whom he or she felt secure.

It is within this context that the conclusions of Gove must be examined in relationship to broadly held First Nations values regarding the role of family in child protection.

Family Conferencing

Family preservation through the use of family-based services developed rapidly in the late 1970s (Nelson and Landsman 1992). Early programs like the St. Paul Family Centered Project through to more recent programs like Homebuilders demonstrated that by providing in home supports, teaching families competencies and emphasizing their strengths, it was possible to protect children. The family and the child's immediate community are viewed as the most valuable resources in the provision of nurture and protection. This approach is regarded as less disruptive to children than the traditional methods of apprehension and placement in foster care. Verna Vaudreuil in her testimony to the Gove Inquiry remembers her own experience of being a child in care when she comments on her first foster home placement by saying, "Mommy and Daddy don't love me any more. I was bad so I got put someplace else" (cited in Gove 1995:14).

Although family-based approaches are an accepted part of child welfare practice, Gove is critical of models that use family group conferencing as an intervention method in child protection. British Columbia's new Child, Family and Community Service Act uses the family group conference as a means to serve the child even after an investigation concludes that a child needs protection (1994 s.20). Gove believes that the family conference approach has several weaknesses, the most important being that it disregards the dynamics of abuse, particularly abuse that is intergenerational. Gove is concerned that the rights and concerns of parents and adult family members may take precedence over the rights of the child and, as a result, children in need of protection may not be able to have their basic needs met within the family.

Developed originally in New Zealand, the family group conference approach has been used extensively with the Maori population of that country. Burford and Pennell (1995) have piloted the method in Newfoundland and Labrador where it has been used with the Inuit of Nain. Gove notes that this approach has been recommended by the Vancouver Regional Child and Youth Committee and by the Community Panel Family and Children's Services Legislation Review. However, a background report for the Gove Inquiry pointed out weaknesses related to the neglect of monitoring and evaluation as well as a disregard for the family dynamics of sexual abuse (Carter 1995). Clearly this concerned Gove and, while he does not reject the concept out of hand, he argues against its use for children who are in need of protection. In Recommendation 85 of his report (Gove 1995:226) he urges the government to amend Section 20 of the Child, Family and Community Service Act by adding "that families in which children are at risk of abuse or neglect are not referred to a family conference." Gove further suggests that the use of the family conference should be discretionary and that the entire concept requires further research and evaluation.

This caution is problematic for First Nations child welfare in that variations of this approach appear to fit well with emerging intervention models used by First Nations. First Nations point out that "children have many mothers" and it is the extended family and community that function as parents. When problems arise it is the community that must take responsibility for its children as opposed to a parent and an agency.

Gove is cautious about the effectiveness of the family group conference model when there is intergenerational abuse. Sexual abuse of children is a problem in First Nations communities and there is not unanimity on how to deal with this issue (Aboriginal Community Panel 1992) which is often intergenerational. However, the approaches which are emerging use the principles of the family group conference within the context of traditional methods like healing and sentencing circles. These emphasize community responsibility in protecting the child through the offender's accountability to the group. Discounting this approach will serve to perpetuate the present system which mitigates against the possibility of reconciliation and holistic healing. It will also undermine the efforts of First Nations people to develop intervention methods that are both culturally appropriate and effective.

Education and Professional Regulation

Gove's recommendations present some logistical and financial challenges for First Nations, especially with the move toward self-government coming at a time when the federal government is making drastic cuts to transfer payments and overall expenditures. The problem in British Columbia is acknowledged by Gove (1995:27) when he points out that federal contributions to BC's social programs will shrink to 11 percent in 1997-98 as a result of the Canada Health and Social Transfer Act. While acknowledging this development, Gove calls for increased competency-based training as well as the bachelor of social work degree as the minimum educational requirement. In British Columbia, as in other provinces, access to education has been an issue for First Nations people. Even in provinces with innovative services, such as the Access Program in Manitoba, First Nations people continue to encounter barriers to post secondary education as the program has been cut to the bone. As the federal government has reduced transfer payments, the Province of Manitoba has reduced funding for this program, requiring students to obtain alternative sources of funding. Treaty status students have had to obtain band sponsorship, in effect off-loading the cost of education from the province to the First Nation.

In British Columbia, education, training and accessibility remain key issues for First Nations. As well the province does not produce enough qualified graduates to meet the demand for Ministry of Social Services child protection workers. Gove indicated that among social workers delivering child protection services in the employ of Ministry of Social Services, 46 percent had no social work education. The remaining 54 percent comprised of 38 percent with a bachelor of social work, nine percent with a master of social work and 7 percent with some amount of social work education below the bachelor degree level. This shortage of qualified social workers is compounded by factors such as high turnover and long periods of probationary employment before workers have full authority to act. Clearly the ministry will continue to have difficulty meeting the education and competence standards suggested by Gove. It will be even more difficult for First Nations to meet these standards as they continue to lack the resources and access to education and training. With many First Nations situated in isolated parts of the province and relying on paraprofessional staff, educating First Nations workers to the bachelor of social work level may prove to be a costly challenge.

The issue of professional regulation is closely connected to education require-ments. Gove has recommended that social workers be registered in order to facilitate regulation of the profession. Regulation is seen as a way to promote greater accountability and a higher standard of practice. Registered social workers are responsible to a board established under provincial legislation. Presently in British Columbia there is a Social Workers Act (1979) that created a Board of Registration, but the Act requires only that social workers engaged in private practice be registered (s.10.11). Gove suggests that all practising social workers should be registered under the Health Professions Act and report to a professional college of social workers.

While some First Nations social workers accept this process of registration, others reject it, seeing it as a means for exerting control over emerging First Nations practice. The idea of regulation creates potential problems in other areas as well. Within First Nations child welfare the community-based approach means that elders and extended family members are integral to intervention and planning. Child welfare committees, or child welfare advisory committees, are made up of lay people, elders and interested community members who are not professionals and who may not have the same view of professional issues like confidentiality. Given the nature of community life, the current code of ethics already presents problems for social workers engaged in northern, rural and remote practice around issues such as dual relationships (Brownlee and Taylor 1995). The code is bound to be even more problematic for workers delivering services to First Nations communities.

This is not to suggest that First Nations (or workers engaged in rural, northern and remote practice for that matter), should reject the principles and ethics of professional social work. Instead it is clear that the profession has to re-examine certain standards and ideals that were developed largely within an urban context of practice. This practice context tends to be one that is specialized and one in which "clients" are not encountered or known outside of the work setting. In First Nations communities the small size and the extended family relationships mean that workers are inextricably bound to the community, creating an entirely different set of practice expectations.

The Question of Aboriginal Ancestry

Gove acknowledges the work and documentation found in *Liberating Our Children: Liberating Our Nations*, but expresses some specific concerns about British Columbia's Child, Family and Community Service Act (1994) as it relates to First Nations children. The test of cultural heritage is considered to be important and Gove makes positive recommendations about speeding up this process in order to arrive more quickly at a plan for children. However, he suggests removing Section 4.2 which states that "If the child is an aboriginal child, the importance of preserving the child's cultural identity must be considered in determining the child's best interests." He reasons that Aboriginal children are already protected under Section 4.1 which states that "all relevant factors must be considered in determining the child's best interests." Under this section "continuity of the child's care" and "the child's cultural, racial, linguistic and religious heritage" are considered fundamental. He further suggests that, by adding Section 4.2, the legislation calls into question the cultural identity of other cultural groups who deserve equal protection for their children.

This view may have legitimacy but raises issues related to special or distinct status for groups in this country, including First Nations. The political leadership of First Nations would argue that distinctions have to be made and the recent agreement with the Nisga'a underlines this point of view. First Nations are distinct and have special status within Canadian confederation. It follows then that legislation should reflect their unique position. This does not diminish or devalue the importance of other cultures within the legislative framework.

Conclusions

Judge Gove has made an important contribution to the development of child welfare services in the Province of British Columbia. The recommendations contained within the report emphasize a view which is child centred. While it was not his intention to make recommendations about the form or substance of First Nations child welfare,[4] the points of view expressed in the report are somewhat narrow and are in conflict with a number of child welfare developments within First Nations. The differences are not irreconcilable and many of Judge Gove's recommendations can be used by First Nations to avoid the mistakes and problems experienced by the Ministry of Social Services in British Columbia. However, approaches to issues such as the protection of children within the context of family and community, professionalization of service, and the distinctiveness of First Nations children will require further exploration and clarification to promote mutual understanding.

Notes

1. A few examples of these provincial inquiries include: Giesbrecht 1992; and Thomlison 1984.
2. Hudson and Taylor-Henley cite Indian and Northern Affairs Canada 1989.
3. Wayne Govereau, an Aboriginal person who was hired as the Child Advocate for Manitoba in 1992 disagreed with Beaulieu's remarks and suggested they misrepresented the contemporary realities.
4. Judge Gove clearly stated this at a public meeting at the Prince George Friendship Centre on May 23, 1996.

Decentralized Social Services and Self-Government: Challenges for First Nations

Diane Gray-Withers

Introduction

Social policies in Canada have largely been developed in national and provincial governmental frameworks, yet their consequences are played out and experienced in local communities (Wharf 1992:20). An ill fit between national policies and the people they are designed to serve is well illustrated at the local level, especially for First Nations people. High levels of unemployment, marked dependencies on income transfers, high suicide rates among First Nations youth, as well as the increasing numbers incarcerated by the justice system are all examples of the inappropriateness of federal and provincial policies to First Nations people.

This chapter proposes that First Nations social problems, with specific regard to child welfare, are best dealt with community members who are capable of ascertaining the local needs and concerns of their people and implementing practical consensual solutions through self-government initiatives. The argument is made that while the delivery of child and family services (CFS) could be more integrated and inclusive under future First Nations self-government, the dual-bilateral and tripartite system of social service policy development and delivery in Manitoba has social, political, jurisdictional and financial problems. These need to be closely examined in order to provide for meaningful community solutions.

A community-based model of government that includes the voices of women in the decision making processes would be one step in acknowledging the important social and political contributions that women have to make. In reviewing some of the current problems of the Native CFS agencies, this chapter suggests that the dominant patriarchal non-Aboriginal culture shapes First Nations leaders' opinions about the role women play in their communities. One result has been a polarization, pitting social concerns against political aspirations.

As a study of the decentralization of social services, the chapter provides a glimpse of some of the problems associated with community delivered child welfare programs. It focuses on the process by which First Nations Child and Family Service Agencies were given the mandate to deliver child welfare services and more specifically on the power struggles that can arise when local governments are given control of implementing social service policy. While some of these problems have been exacerbated by the political struggle First Nations communities face in striving toward self-government, it is worthwhile to examine these issues.

First Nations Women and Self-Government

Since the early 1980s, social services in Manitoba have undergone a transformation with regard to First Nations children. Significant concern was displayed over the high number of Native children removed from their homes and placed in white foster care or adopted into white homes in what has now been referred to as the "sixties sweep" (First Nations Child and Family Task Force 1993:15). The response to the outrage and politicization of these events by Native women's groups was the decentralization of child and family services in the early 1980s and the creation of regional Native Child and Family Service agencies. Tripartite or dual-bilateral agreements[1] were drawn up between the federal government, provincial government and First Nations communities, giving these agencies the mandate to provide child and family services in their geographical jurisdictions.[2] The perceived solution to the problems that contributed to the cultural genocide of First Nations was the implementation of provincial social policies by First Nations regional agencies.

These political and social changes have often been considered a part of the larger project for First Nations self-government in Manitoba. In addressing the need for community development initiatives, this chapter will discuss a few of the pressing issues which surround the current system of First Nations delivery of child and family services and note how certain problems could be intensified or resolved through true self-government in Manitoba.

Particular attention will be paid to the concerns of First Nations women that have been expressed through interviews conducted in research for this chapter.[3] To date, there has been little credence or academic attention paid to First Nations women's control over social services or input into self-government initiatives. Native women's groups have been vocal in their criticism of self-government where it entails the further domination of First Nations men over the lives of women and children.[4] They want the opportunity to balance the social requirements of their families and the politics of self-government.[5]

Over the last few years in Manitoba close attention has been paid to issues surrounding the dismantling of Department of Indian Affairs and Northern Development (DIAND) and the restoration of jurisdictions through First Nations self-government. This focus is understandable, given the importance of the agreements. Nevertheless, it has shifted attention away from other worthy issues, some of which are critical for true self-determination. These areas include CFS and the development and delivery of other social services in First Nations communities.

The Dismantling of the Department of Indian Affairs and Northern Development

The concept of self-government emerges from Native history and aspirations. Native peoples have a unique political and constitutional position, "yet they recognize that their marginality can only be dealt with by capturing a degree of political power which hitherto has been denied them" (Loxley 1981:162). Throughout the period of political and administrative subordination to the federal government, First Nations have retained strong memories of political independence; moreover, the bitter experiences of colonialism have kept alive in their souls a vision of self-determination—a sovereign government by their people (Boldt 1993:87-88). The claim for self-government is that it is an inherent right, pre-dating the arrival of Europeans and the cultural, political and economic domination that followed.

For First Nations people, the "self" in self-government means more than delivering programs and administering policies designed by other governments and non-Aboriginal people (Winnipeg Council of First Nations 1994:18).[6] It means defining, through the practice of policy development and implementation, how First Nations governments can be used to come to terms with important problems and objectives in Native communities (Cassidy 1990:80). To administer the programs as designed and financed through a residual model of social welfare is to merely replace the existing non-Aboriginal Department of Indian Affairs with a Native one.[7] There is a need to move away from the paternalism of the current system to support for First Nations self-government (Mercredi 1991:4, 5, 8). According to the director of Ma Mawi Wi Chi Itata Centre, George Munroe, the dismantling process also means empowering the people in communities to take control over their communities' problems and find solutions.[8] It means giving women and children a voice in the development process.

Morrissette et al. (1993:94) argue that the process of colonization involves creating dependency. This is accomplished through: structural measures such as removing Aboriginal people from their land through treaties and the implementation of a reserve system; cultural measures such as displacement of traditional forms of governance with representative democracy and an authoritarian model of leadership; social and economic measures such as the creation of a welfare economy; and the devaluation of traditional spirituality and knowledge through the residential school system, the health system and the child welfare system.

During the course of economic and political development in Manitoba, the foreign "white" system imposed itself on the Native economy. The sociopolitical culture, as determined by non-Native political structures and economic activities, became the basis of colonialism and colonial relations (Bourgeault 1983:50). The colonial exploitation of Native society over the years resulted in a transformation of the social relationships that caused the subjugation of First Nations women. First Nations men in Manitoba became responsible for the production of commodities in the fur trade and the development of mercantile capitalism and, in doing so, assumed the role as provider of the family. First Nations women were thus encouraged and even forced to become dependent upon men (Bourgeault 1983:55). The Indigenous Women's Collective of Manitoba noted in its *Report on the Discussion of the Inherent Right to Self-Government* that:

> the role of the political order of European societies lay in the positions held by men who owned property, and their ability to generate a strong financial position for themselves. This role did not require the involvement of women. In fact, women and children were considered part of the property held by men. (1994:6)

Morrissette et al. (1993) make the connection between the colonization policies of the Canadian government on First Nations people and the adoption of a colonial attitude among elements of the Aboriginal community itself. They state that "this [has] contributed to the high level of internalized violence within Aboriginal communities, particularly against women and children, and the failure of Aboriginal leaders to address this issue adequately" (1993:94). First Nations women are not only battling the non-Native society for respect and recognition of their concerns, they also fight for these issues with men in their own communities.

While Morrissette and his colleagues develop an understanding of colonialization and its impact upon First Nations communities, they do not address the patriarchal overtones that are both implicit and explicit in policies such as the Indian Act and the effects that these influences have had upon First Nations men and their attitudes towards women. Sections of the Indian Act continue to refuse women the right to own reserve housing or property. By assigning a male as head of the household, the Act naturally subordinates the woman and makes her dependent upon a man for subsistence. As Pateman (1989:132) argues, "Women have never been completely excluded from public life; but, the way in which women are included is grounded, as firmly as their position in the domestic sphere, in patriarchal beliefs and practices."[9]

The band councils and Indian government structures are creations of the federal government established for the purpose of administering federal transfers and programs. These structures are completely rooted in the colonial and patriarchal traditions of the Indian Act, and generally serve to exclude women from having a political voice within their communities. The conditions of unrestrained power was engendered by generations of colonialism, the Indian Agent and the Indian Act. When the Indian Agents left communities, many First Nations leaders were thrust into positions of power within their communities and nations with a virtual blank cheque on decision making in the community (Wastasecoot 1995:2).

John Loxley, in "The Great Northern Plan" (1981), discusses the replacement of the Indian Agent by Native federal employees. By virtue of their new role, the Native employees occupy a contradictory position within their communities. They are mainly male and hold positions of authority as granted by the federal government, but they are not policy makers. The contradictory pressures of the state's desire for accountability and the communities' need for more flexibility in policies and financial spending places these people in a nebulous position. They may be considered part of a neocolonialist agenda because they are responsible for the implementation of state policies and programs, while they also struggle to appear responsive to their own communities.

In many communities, the male-dominated Native leadership has hidden and perpetuated problems of child abuse (Rider 1992:5).[10] In order for problems of violence and abuse to be addressed at a community level, a zero tolerance policy on violence must be adopted by the Chiefs and councillors. Sharon Carstairs, former Liberal Party leader of Manitoba, stated that "the Assembly of Manitoba Chiefs (AMC) has got to be more open about what is happening on reserves. Collective rights end up being only the rights of its male members" (Teichroeb 1992). It is not enough to simply restore jurisdictional authority to First Nations governments. A process of empowerment for women and their communities will need to occur to allow for true community development and the acceptance of responsibility for current problems. While these problems have been the result of policies of paternalism, subordination and colonialism, all community members need to work together to ascertain solutions that will help communities and people to heal.

The restoration of jurisdictions to First Nations is, in essence, a political step towards self-government. The Framework Agreement, signed on December 7, 1994, occurred with the objective of establishing a formal, binding process between the minister (DIAND) and the Assembly of Manitoba Chiefs for the purpose of restoring to First Nations governments the jurisdictions consistent with the inherent right to self-government.[11] The dismantling of DIAND is symbolically important for the communities and the AMC. It entails transferring complete administrative control from the federal government to the communities. However, for the Chief and councillors in First Nations communities to be more than administrators of other governments' policies, they need the authority to pass their own laws and policies within their jurisdictions. Furthermore, the political symbolism of the dismantling process needs to be juxtaposed against the patriarchal systems existing in many communities, where it is commonplace for political agendas, to interfere in social concerns and affairs.[12]

It is the lived reality of First Nations women that they, more so than the men in their communities, are involved with local and provincial authorities whose jurisdictions include health, education and child welfare.[13] Not only have these areas been perceived by the political leadership in provincial and federal governmental structures as appropriate for women, it has enforced a structural reality on the role First Nations women play in their own communities. These social responsibilities typically are devalued and hidden in the process of negotiating self-government. Kathleen Jamieson (1979) has articulated that First Nations women experience multiple jeopardy: they are women and they are Native. They not only face white male governments but also male-dominated Native organizations (Jamieson 1979:157-78). For women to have a role in self-government and for communities to be truly involved in development initiatives, they need to free themselves from the social–political division that has been imposed upon them by a colonist society and work to overcome this dichotomy. The political relevance of social considerations must be recognized. Similarly, women need to be perceived as having an important role to play in community development and be accorded equality in treatment and attitudes.[14]

The Current Child Welfare System

This section reviews some of the problems that are inherent in the current Native child welfare system in Manitoba. Unresolved constitutional and jurisdictional issues are overriding concerns. These include the federal government's devolution of responsibilities to the province for standards' maintenance and child welfare policy development, and arguments over who is ultimately responsible for First Nations families and children. Obviously, the objective of self-government is to resolve these constitutional and jurisdictional issues. What this essentially means is that the current jurisdictional wars will be resolved when First Nations regain control and authority over their own lives.

The federal government has consistently refused to pass Indian child welfare legislation, yet it still retains exclusive constitutional authority to enact legislation with respect to First Nations. Section 91 (24) of the Constitution Act of 1867, gives exclusive legislative authority for Indians and lands reserved for Indians to the federal government, and the federal government has used this in the past to enact The Indian Act. This relationship was also referred to in Section 35 of the Constitution Act of 1982, which affirmed Aboriginal and treaty rights. The Indian Act, with the exception of education and limited health regulations, is silent on social services. Section 88 permits provincial laws of general application to apply to Indians on reserves, unless these laws are inconsistent with federal legislation. Provinces legislate under Section 92(13) of the Constitution Act of 1867, which sets out the provinces' exclusive jurisdiction in property and civil rights. Although the federal government has the constitutional authority to enact specific legislation in Indian child welfare matters, it chooses not to do so as child welfare is considered to be a provincial responsibility. The policy of the Department of Indian Affairs has been to secure agreements with the provinces and the territories to deliver child welfare services on reserves (Pimento 1985:1).

While the provincial government is responsible for service standards with regard to First Nations child welfare, the federal government provides the financial support for child welfare in First Nations communities. The provinces and the federal government currently do not agree over which level of government is responsible for funding child welfare initiatives for First Nations families off-reserve.[15] Until April 1996, child welfare was provided primarily by the provincial government, but cost shared with the federal government through the Canada Assistance Plan. Through the Canada Health and Social Transfer, implemented in April 1996, the province now receives block funding from the federal government for its social programs.[16] Chief Dennis Pashe notes "that the lack of resources and services . . . is the result of a game of political football played between the federal and provincial governments" (1995:A7).

The jurisdictional complexities surrounding the provision of social services to First Nations peoples have resulted in the fragmentation of many programs. The federal position that services and programs for Natives residing in First Nations communities must be accommodated within existing federal–provincial jurisdictional arrangements and practices has resulted in gaps in programs and services. With regard to child welfare, provinces have enforced their statutes in such matters as custody and removal of children from First Nations communities, while non-statutory services, such as counselling and family support, have been available inconsistently to families who live in First Nations communities (Schaan 1994:114). Further problems have arisen because Ottawa and the Province of Manitoba both refuse to assume financial responsibility for non-mandated services in the communities. While there is adequate funding for crisis intervention into families, there is little or no funding for prevention-related activities.[17]

Federal preference has been for the delivery of social services through institutions accredited under provincial jurisdiction or to provincial standards as is the case with child welfare (Schaan 1994:114).[18] The approach developed in Manitoba requires that First Nations regional agencies meet the province's service delivery standards and implement provincial child welfare policies. Native agencies are incorporated through agreements with the province and the federal government that are either tripartite or dual-bilateral.

While tripartite or dual-bilateral agreements are required in the existing legislation, they are not actually the incorporating instruments.[19] An order-in-council and a subsequent schedule allows the minister of Family Services with the approval of Cabinet, to enter into agreements with Native bands or tribal councils to incorporate the band or council to become an agency and provide services under the Child Welfare Act. Although the schedule allows for individual bands to form child welfare agencies, the province prefers to sign with tribal councils.[20] The provincial rationale behind not mandating individual bands to implement provincial child welfare practices is that there is more service accountability, policy coordination and economy of scale with regional boards.[21] Currently, seven regional agencies exist in the province of Manitoba: Cree Child and Family Caring Agency; Awasis; West Region; Anishinaabe;

Intertribal; South-East; and Dakota Ojibwa.

Jurisdiction is used by the provincial government to define the geographical area for which CFS agencies are mandated. CFS agencies use the term to denote First Nations claims for service provision for its membership for the purpose of administering the child protection mandate (Hudson and Taylor-Henley 1993:51). The current system, while an improvement over the former white, centralized CFS system, should not be taken as a concrete example of First Nations self-government. The policies are designed by the government of Manitoba even though they do allow for some cultural flexibility. In the current system, accountability is directed to the government, not to the people in the communities. With a primary financial focus on intervention, there is neither adequate flexibility nor finances to develop more holistic and culturally appropriate practices.

Three separate inquiries into First Nations child welfare have recently come to light. The Aboriginal Justice Inquiry (Manitoba, Government of 1991), the Desjarlais Inquest ((Manitoba, Government of 1992) and the First Nations Child and Family Task Force ((Manitoba, Government of 1993) all examined the Native child welfare system and produced reports that differed in their treatment of the subject. The Aboriginal Justice Inquiry and the First Nations Child and Family Task Force both recommended that increased decentralization and further moves towards First Nations self-government were necessary to deal with the underlying causes of violence, abuse and neglect in Aboriginal society. The Desjarlais Inquest, however, recommended that further accountability and centralization was necessary for protection of First Nations children.

Georgina Crate, director of Intertribal Child and Family Service Agency, noted that there must be responsibility, ownership and accountability for and by First Nations for the quality of care, policies and standards that are provided (1992:23). Only through community accountability and the desire to address problems such as violence and abuse can healing begin. Policy development by the provincial government, along with centralization and strict accountability, was not effective in solving child welfare problems. There is no indication that returning Native child welfare to a centralized, strictly controlled environment would solve the problems that are inherent in the system. Therefore, while accountability and political interference are both problems under the current provincial child welfare system, the process of empowering communities through self-government to address problems by designing programs and policies that meet their needs may be a more effective way of ensuring ownership and accountability for the system.

The second problem that has arisen in the Native CFS agencies is the conflict between the regional offices and local control by the Chiefs.[22] Tensions occur when individual bands demand control of CFS in their own communities yet the regional office wants central control for reasons of accountability—both in terms of policy implementation and financial responsibility. This pull between centralization and decentralization has led to claims of political interference in social services and direct conflicts of interest. Criticisms have been voiced by Aboriginal women's groups both on- and off-reserve that First Nations leadership has emphasized political goals at the expense of service goals. They fear that the achievement of self-government would continue to concentrate power in the hands of the Chiefs—who are predominately male (Hudson and Taylor-Henley 1993:52). The point emphasized by these women was that they favoured regional control of child welfare, which would hopefully offset the domination of the Chiefs in local social matters.[23]

The following events which occurred in Manitoba in 1992 underscored the notion of a centralization–decentralization conundrum.[24] Because some children in care had died, while others had been allegedly left or placed in potentially abusive homes, Aboriginal women's groups and the province publicly accused some Chiefs of complicity and political self-serving interference. The Chiefs responded by accusing the province of ulterior motives, specifically for attempting to discredit aspirations for self-government. One of the Aboriginal women's groups publicly expressed its doubts about self-government and whether or not women and children would be protected by it (Hudson and Taylor-Henley 1993:54).

This situation underlines the battle that First Nations women face. The concern of the Chiefs was saving face and avoiding political embarrassment. Choices were made within communities that were political in nature; the Chief or band council interfered in social decision making processes by insisting that children remain in potentially abusive situations because of whom the child was related to.[25]

First Nations women continue to struggle against patriarchal structures in government, in their own communities and in society. First Nations women have successfully fought against aspects of the patriarchal Indian Act and, with Bill C-31, won the right to keep or regain (if previously lost) their Indian status.[26] Yet other parts of the Indian Act still remain extraordinarily patriarchal—with men being the owners of the property and houses in most communities. The Chiefs and other men in the communities who support political goals over social goals reinforce the divisions between men and women. Ultimately, there is a dichotomy between the First Nations women who struggle for social goals and service provision and men who desire to achieve political self-government. Unless these two elements can be successfully accommodated, there will be no unity in the political fight to secure self-determination.

George Munroe[27] has noted that Aboriginal women do have a valid concern in fearing that certain Chiefs will utilize the political mechanism of self-government to increase their own personal power. However, he worries that divide and conquer techniques have been successful in separating the Aboriginal community. Communities must join their social ("low road") and political ("high road") forces to provide for meaningful change and achieve self-government (Hudson and Taylor-Henley 1993:54).

While there is a need to unite the political and the social in terms of self-determination and accord social goals greater respect, social policy must also be kept appropriately separated from political aspirations for women to feel powerful and comfortable in their own communities.[28] The patriarchal Indian Act and the dominant white culture have been instrumental in reshaping Native attitudes towards women and the role they play in their communities. As in the non-Aboriginal society, the power of the political orders came to lie with men, leaving women and children to be considered the property of men. The colonization processes undertaken by policies of the Canadian government have caused discord, adversarial attitudes and dysfunctional communities.

For women to feel secure under self-government, their voices need to be included. The current band council system is an extension of DIAND to which the Chief and council are responsible (Indigenous Women's Collective 1993:27). Many women are concerned that the "restoration of jurisdictions" will merely concentrate more power in the hands of a few Chiefs. This could have a further negative impact on their lives and the lives of their children. The establishment of a Women's Directorate, as advocated by the Indigenous Women's Collective, may allow First Nations women participation in self-government initiatives (Indigenous Women's Collective 1994:44-48).The directorate could be designed to ensure the active involvement of First Nations women, both on- and off-reserve, in all matters directly affecting them. If accorded input equal to the Assembly of Manitoba Chiefs on both political self-government and community development initiatives, it would involve First Nations women in the decision making process and encourage political accountability and participation in self-government.

Accountability to an authority above the community political leadership must be developed both in terms of self-government and current child welfare programs. The Cree Nation Child and Family Caring Agency, Manitoba's newest agency (1993), built into their tripartite agreement the mandatory exclusion of the Chiefs and the band councillors from the regional authority. South-East Child and Family Services has also developed policies that prevent the Chief or members of the council from sitting on the board of the agency. These two agencies are the exceptions, however. Other agencies, such as Anishinaabe and Intertribal, have publicly declared that political interference has caused conflicts of interest. The Dakota Ojibway Child and Family Services was singled out in the Desjarlais Inquest (Manitoba, Government of 1992) as requiring the separation of politics from its social agenda. Native women's groups and the First Nation's Child and Family Task Force (Manitoba, Government of 1993) indicated that a separate, autonomous board composed of impartial representatives should be established to act as an appeal mechanism when conflicts occur in agencies.

The final challenge for child and family service provision under self-government is the need to develop a practice for urban areas.[29] Rosalee Tizya, in "Aboriginal Governments and Power Sharing in Canada" (1992), notes that the Indian Act system has left off-reserve Natives dangling between the jurisdictions of the federal and provincial governments. The federal government has limited its responsibility to on-reserve Indians, but the provincial government has argued that all Aboriginal peoples are a federal responsibility (Tizya 1992:21). While child welfare agencies operate in a defined geographical area, several First Nations CFS agencies feel that they should be allowed to operate on an outreach basis in urban centres. Yet, other urban social agencies want a mandate to provide an increased spectrum of services to all Aboriginal people, regardless of their status.[30] The requirement for intervention in CFS cases continues to pose a geographical problem.[31] The current urban agencies are not mandated by the province and provide voluntary services in a "status blind" manner.

Will urban Native CFS agencies have to be devised to overlap with the current non-Aboriginal CFS authorities or will existing CFS agencies have their mandate expanded to allow them to operate in an outreach capacity to off-reserve members? Native CFS agencies have attempted to extend their mandate to off-reserve members in the past, causing conflict with provincial CFS agencies. For example, one case concerning outreach services referred to provincial court in 1991 concluded that the current child welfare legislation does not legally extend Native agencies' mandate off-reserve (Olijnyk 1991:1, 5). Because many First Nations people residing in Winnipeg or other areas of the province, do not belong to a specific community in the province, an urban Native child welfare agency would need to be created to provide child welfare to families off-reserve. This new agency, would have to define exactly who would be eligible to receive their services. Would eligibility apply to status Indians or would child welfare services be provided on a status-blind basis?

Conclusions

The federal government now actively recognizes First Nations self-government and has devolved 85 percent of its administrative authority in areas such as education, social assistance, and child and family services to First Nations communities and agencies.[32] These measures need to be accompanied by steps to provide for autonomy with regard to CFS and alternative approaches to social assistance, both of which are tied intrinsically and holistically to the social and political components of self-determination.

Will the dismantling process create true self-determination and afford First Nations communities the ability to take control of community development? The federal government is very anxious to restore jurisdiction to First Nations. Concerns have been raised that this may be the foreshadowing of an off-loading of fiscal responsibility. The federal government, since the 1980s, has been slowly cutting programs and services and many people believe that the economic and social situations in many communities will get worse before community development initiatives have any impact upon the problems.[33]

The dismantling process is being positively received by the federal government because it may be able to relieve itself of long term financial responsibility to the communities—most of which are suffering from poor housing, inadequate hospitals and educational facilities, and basic amenities such as running water or electricity. The transfer of responsibility would leave Ottawa appearing less politically accountable for First Nations people and communities. Greater local control will result in Native people in control of their own futures but, unless funding levels are stabilized or increased, the restoration of jurisdictions may worsen current circumstances (Angus 1991:27). Furthermore, there is rampant corruption and nepotism in many communities—a sentiment echoed by all the women interviewed. The Chiefs concerned have a political power that is seldom challenged. Women do not want this type of unaccountable, corrupt patriarchy to be given even more power through self-government.

In many First Nations communities people still react with fear to the suggestion of self-government, not because they do not understand what it means, but because they fear the consequences of greater power being concentrated in the hands of one or a few people in their Nations under present conditions (Wastasecoot 1995:2). Women have been side-lined, dependent upon the Chiefs for determining whether they will get housing, or even whether they or another family member will be employed in one of the few positions available in the communities. Their lack of control is reflective of the lack of control First Nations people have had over their lives for 125 years. The patriarchal community structures have been established and encouraged by the dominant white political culture for the administration of treaty lands and do not constitute traditional political cultures or norms. The result has been the pitting of women and their social concerns against men and their political aspirations. There is a real need for these social and political goals to meet and work together for community development.

Community oriented and decentralized social services have the greatest potential for addressing problems common to the delivery of child and family services. However, only an emphasis on participatory democracy, which integrates the communities' social and political goals, can allow for increased accountability in the communities (McKenzie 1994b:106). If this condition is not met, self-government will fail to adequately address many of the problems of the system it hopes to replace (McKenzie 1994b:108). The first priority of First Nations leaders should be to build viable communities that will enable policy making to address the inherent problems in child welfare administration (Indigenous Women's Collective 1994:39).

Notes

1. Agreements signed with First Nations Regional Agencies have generally taken the form of a tripartite agreement involving the federal government, the provincial government and the First Nations Tribal Council. In the early 1980s, before this policy was established, the Dakota Ojibway Tribal Council entered into two complementary but separate bilateral agreements with the province of Manitoba and the federal government. Thus, the term "dual-bilateral" was established to refer to this form of agreement.

2. The one exception to this rule has been the Sagkeeng First Nation which has been practising non-mandated child and family services to the community of Fort Alexander since the 1970s and falls under the authority of the Eastman provincial regional office (a non-native CFS regional office).

3. The author interviewed twenty-two First Nations women from a variety of First Nations communities. Their names have not been included in the bibliography to protect their anonymity. Throughout the next, the interviews will be referred to numerically.

4. Personal interview with Kathy Mallett, Director of the Original Women's Network of Winnipeg, January 13, 1995.

5. Interviews 1-20 with First Nations women.

6. This paper notes that the mere dismantling of Indian Affairs and systems would not be "self-government" per se, but rather "self-administration."

7. In "Alternatives to Social Assistance in Indian Communities" (Mercredi 1991:4), there is the assertion that programs currently in place serving First Nations are based on the residual model of social welfare, which is the dominant one in Canadian society. The model is keyed to the administration of individualized social assistance transfers to people who have failed for whatever reasons to meet the minimal demands of the market. The interventionist policies designed by the provincial government with regard to child welfare have been constructed in a similar fashion. The situations that warranted intervention in the past ended with children being removed, not just from homes, but from entire communities. As with social assistance, First Nations have asserted that these measures are completely culturally inappropriate and have demanded that a more holistic, community-based approach be adopted.

8. Personal interview with George Munroe, Director of Ma Mawi, Winnipeg, February 15, 1995.

9. Carol Pateman's book, *The Disorder of Women* (1989:123), develops the theory of the universal dichotomy between private and public in civil society itself.

10. Discussed in interviews with Kathy Mallett, Director of the Original Women's Network (est. 1995), and social workers from Anishinaabe Child and Family Services and West Region Child and Family Services (est. 1995).

11. See Assembly of Manitoba Chiefs, *Framework Agreement: The Dismantling of DIAND, the Restoration of Jurisdictions to First Nations Peoples in Manitoba and Recognition of First Nations Governments in Manitoba*, Winnipeg: Assembly of Manitoba Chiefs, December 7, 1994.

12. Expressed in interviews 1-16; 19-22.

13. Expressed in all twenty-two interviews.

14. A report by the Indigenous Women's Collective of Manitoba Inc. (1993) provides a synopsis of indigenous women's viewpoints on self-government and other

initiatives.

15. Since 1993, when the federal government ended its reimbursement of provincial expenditures for social services for Aboriginal people living off-reserve, it is estimated that the cost to Manitoba for social assistance alone has exceeded $100 million.

16. The fiscal reductions in Manitoba that accompany the Canada Health and Social Transfer are expected to amount to $277 million by the year 2000.

17. In 1996, the federal government discontinued funding to the First Nations child and family services agencies for Services to Families programming. The funding cut will severely impact First Nations agencies' capacity to deliver preventative services. Ironically, the annual budget of $2.2 million for Services to Families was less than the savings in child maintenance expenditures that the agencies have achieved in the past few years through the use of preventative family support services.

18. Also see *Native People in Canada: Contemporary Conflicts* (Frideres 1988:260-95).

19. Manitoba, Government of. *The Child and Family Services Act*, outlines the agencies incorporated to fulfil the provincial child welfare mandate.

20. The one exception to this was the creation of Awasis which involved three tribal councils and three independent First Nations communities.

21. Personal interview with senior provincial civil servant, Department of Family Services, Province of Manitoba, February 13, 1995.

22. Expressed by all First Nations women in interviews 1-22.

23. Interviews 3-5; 7-18; 21-22.

24. This phrase is used by Peter Aucoin and Herman Bakvis (1988) in their book *The Centralization–Decentralization Conundrum: Organization and Management in the Canadian Government.*

25. Interview with Kathy Mallett, Director of the Original Women's Network, January 13, 1995; social worker from West Region Child and Family Services, February 14, 1995; and interviews 6, 12 and 14 with First Nations women.

26. For more information on this, see *Enough is Enough: Aboriginal Women Speak Out*, as told to Janet Silman (Toronto: Women's Press 1987). Bill C-31 is an amendment to the Indian Act which allows First Nations women and children to regain their status previously lost through marriage to a non-status man.

27. Personal interview, George Munroe, February 15, 1995.

28. Interviews 1-8; 11-18; 21 and 22.

29. The Aboriginal Justice Inquiry states that there are approximately 32,000 Treaty Indians in Winnipeg. Census Canada estimates this figure to be 45,000 (Editorial, *Winnipeg Free Press,* June 13, 1994).

30. Personal interview, Wayne Helgason, Executive Director of Winnipeg Social Planning Council, President of National Association of Friendship Centres, January 20, 1995.

31. A report published by the Indigenous Women's Collective (1993:25) discusses the fact that, for women living off-reserve, the issue of self-government is more complex in terms of jurisdictional debates (for example, child welfare issues, etc.) than it is for women living on-reserve.

32. Personal interview, Grand Chief Phil Fontaine of the Assembly of Manitoba Chiefs, February 24, 1995.

33. *And the Last Shall Be First: Native Policy in an Era of Cutbacks* (Angus 1991:23) poses that Native people inevitably will be among the victims of any cuts in government spending because they are already a marginalized group in Canadian society—demographically, regionally, economically, politically and racially.

Connecting Policy and Practice in First Nations Child and Family Services: A Manitoba Case Study

BRAD MCKENZIE[1]

This chapter is based on a case study of the West Region Child and Family Services (CFS), a child welfare agency serving nine First Nations communities in western Manitoba. The agency, governed by a board of Chiefs from the West Region Tribal Council, began operation in 1982 and received its mandate as a child caring agency under provincial legislation in 1985. A decentralized, community-based model of child and family services has been in place for First Nations in Manitoba since the early 1980s, and agencies, organized within Tribal Council areas, operate under a delegated model of authority which includes federal funding for most services, provincial responsibility for legislation and standards, and First Nations control over administration and service delivery.

Factors which influenced First Nations control over child welfare in Manitoba and elsewhere have been well documented (Johnston 1983; McKenzie and Hudson 1985; Kimelman 1985). These include the over-representation of Aboriginal children in care, and the assimilative nature of conventional approaches to intervention. Conventional child welfare services have been correctly characterized as an extension of the colonization process because they devalued Aboriginal family structure, culture and community and played a major role in the removal and often permanent cross cultural placement of Aboriginal children (McKenzie and Hudson 1985; Aboriginal Community Panel 1992; Armitage 1993a). Delegated authority for the delivery of services is one expression of the right to self-government (Taylor-Henley and Hudson 1992), and this general policy direction is now relatively well established for First Nations people living on reserves.

This case study is best described as policy evaluation research, and such studies can be distinguished by the scope of the policy being addressed. Wharf and Callahan (1984) identify four levels: societal/federal; service sector or field of practice; organizational; and the practice arena. The focus of this research is the organizational or agency level. However, the interplay between different levels of policy development require one to consider issues beyond the organizational context, and these relationships are examined where appropriate.

A First Nations organizational emphasis has been chosen for two reasons.

First, it is at the organizational level that the connections between policy and practice take on new meaning as staff struggle to translate general principles and goals into services which affect the well-being of individuals, families and communities. Second, there are few assessments of service delivery processes and outcomes within the field of First Nations child and family services. Most analyses of First Nations Child and Family Services (CFS) (see Aboriginal Community Panel 1992; First Nations Child and Family Task Force 1993) focus on macro-level issues, including the impact of colonization, and propose general models and methods for intervention. While evaluation studies of some First Nations agencies in Manitoba have been conducted (Hudson and McKenzie 1984; Coopers and Lybrand Consulting Group 1987; Hudson and Taylor-Henley 1987a) these are limited by their attention to the early implementation phase of First Nations control over CFS. Indeed, the devolution of such services is relatively recent; thus, the feasibility of assessing service models and their impact over time is only beginning to be explored.

There are a number of frameworks which can be utilized for assessing policy development, but Moroney (1981) has proposed a value-analytic approach that is organized as a three part model. This model includes a policy analysis stage, a program development stage and a program evaluation stage. At the policy analysis stage consideration is given to problem analysis, the specification of value criteria to be used in strategy selection, generation and review of alternate strategies and choice of strategies. Phases of the program development stage include the specification of program objectives, the development of implementation criteria, program design and implementation, whereas evaluation includes monitoring, evaluation and feedback. It is a general model but its primary advantage in First Nations policy assessment is the attention paid to the selection of appropriate value criteria which shape one's understanding of the problem, goal selection and strategy choice. Thus, this model can incorporate the utilization of "inside" knowledge and understanding, including an appreciation of conventional child welfare services as an agent of colonization in First Nations, and the adoption of value criteria such as culturally appropriate services and community control as a means to empowerment. While this framework provides a general guide, more detailed operational issues must also be examined, particularly when completing a post-hoc policy assessment of an agency. Flynn (1992) provides more specific guidance in his outline of the key factors to be included in content and process approaches to agency policy analysis. Of particular importance to the present study are variables associated with system functioning, resource analysis and the impact of the policy or program on selected consumer values, including effectiveness, service responsiveness and rights.

Policy Context and Strategic Issues

In Manitoba, three general policy issues have been important in First Nations CFS. These include: the number of First Nations children in care; service quality concerns within some First Nations agencies, including concerns about political interference at the local community level; and the incorporation of traditional cultural values and practices within a service model which must also ensure the protection of children at risk.

The over-representation of Aboriginal children in care has been attributed to the interventionist role of conventional child welfare authorities (Dumont 1988; Aboriginal Community Panel 1992; First Nations Child and Family Task Force 1993). However, the evolution of First Nations control over service delivery has not led to a reversal of this trend even though children in alternate care may now be in more community-based, culturally appropriate placements. For example, between 1987 and 1990, a 30 percent increase in children in care was reported by First Nations agencies in Manitoba (BDO Ward Mallette 1991:28). In fact, this trend should not be surprising. The lack of child welfare services on reserves prior to the 1980s, recognition of the extent of physical and sexual abuse in First Nations communities, poor economic and social conditions, limited funding for prevention, the lack of complementary social services, the intergenerational impact of the residential school system, and the relatively recent adoption of a community-based service model contribute to the demand for crisis oriented services and higher rates of children in care.

Service quality concerns and the impact of political interference are two closely related issues. Urban-based Aboriginal women's groups were the first to publicly express concerns about the impact of political interference by First Nations community leaders concerning services provided to women and children. Allegations of abuse cover-ups and the protection of relatives were highlighted in a 1992 inquest into the suicide of an adolescent in the care of Dakota Ojibwa Child and Family Services (Giesbrecht 1992). This concern is not confined to Manitoba. For example, Wayne Christian, former Chief of the Spallumcheen First Nation in British Columbia, has observed that personality and politics can be barriers to quality services at the community level. Although an advocate of local autonomy, Christian (1994) argues that community jurisdiction over services and standards carries an obligation that the rights and needs of children be placed above politics. In Manitoba, conflict of interest guidelines and procedures have been developed, although they have yet to be adopted by all First Nations CFS agencies. While political interference remains problematic in some communities, increased awareness of this issue has led to a reduction in the number of complaints about local political interference in investigation and case management decision making. Service quality concerns have also been associated with the level of staff training and the accessibility of specialized assessment and treatment services. These are being generally addressed through a focus on staff training, including distance delivery of the bachelor of social work program from the University of Manitoba, and the development of a wider range of community-based service responses.

A third issue is the recognized need to incorporate culturally appropriate services and standards within a child welfare service model which has been borrowed from conventional residual welfare theory, and is reinforced by existing legislation, standards and funding arrangements. The issue of jurisdictional control is closely related to the development of culturally specific services. Provincial jurisdiction over legislation, standards and related requirements for accountability remain contentious issues. Indeed, the initial acceptance of these arrangements by Manitoba First Nations has always been regarded as an interim measure, and the longer term goal of distinct standards and legislation remains an important priority.

Jurisdictional control is an essential component of self-government, and there is evidence that it is associated with the development of more culturally appropriate services, including the number of Aboriginal foster care providers (McKenzie 1995). It is also important to recognize that control over child and family policy and services is more than simply a political aspiration. For most Aboriginal people it is a profoundly personal issue because they have experienced the loss of family members to a system that has been unconcerned historically about the importance of cultural and family connections. While these arguments support greater autonomy, the limits of localization and the need for checks and balances must be recognized. For example, in some Manitoba communities the goal of local autonomy has been pursued without adequate assurance of the community's capacity to respond to the complexity of needs within families and to guarantee children a basic right to protection.

The issue of culturally appropriate services is also complicated. The concept "culturally appropriate" has become so widely used in relation to Aboriginal services that it is difficult to ascribe any common meaning to it. Variations among Aboriginal people in their identification with traditional culture are recognized, and this has an effect in determining what culturally appropriate services mean to them. Morrissette (1991) describes these as perspectives along a continuum which include traditional, neotraditional and non-traditional beliefs and practices. At the traditional end of the continuum, Aboriginal people adhere to the teachings of the elders, ancestral values and a symbiotic relationship with the environment. Moreover, with the revitalization of early spiritual practices, a growing number of Aboriginal people are incorporating more traditional practices in their lives. Some Aboriginal people can be identified as neotraditional in that they identify with a blend of spirituality and practices that reflect both indigenous beliefs and those values emerging from the dominant society. At the other end of the continuum is a category that includes those who adopt a non-traditional lifestyle. While this group may be less likely to adopt traditional values and customs it cannot be assumed that this will always be the case. This framework implies that culturally appropriate services which affect an individual should respect that person's relative identification with traditional values and customs.

While this principle may be adopted in providing services to individuals, there are also general differences among communities, nations and communities within nations that need to be respected. Of particular significance is the relative impact of the dominant culture and Christianity in shaping the norms and practices within specific communities. This reality and the need to empower local communities require that the development of culturally appropriate policies incorporate a community-based approach which begins with an understanding of local values and practices.

Although Aboriginal people do not embrace a single philosophy, fundamental differences in the world views between the dominant euro-Canadian and Aboriginal cultures are generally acknowledged. Aboriginal cultures typically adopt a more communal approach to helping, group and family reciprocity, a more holistic relationship with nature and other persons, and they value the importance of traditional spirituality, elders and the extended family or clan system (Hamilton and Sinclair 1991; Red Horse 1980; Clarkson, Morrissette and Regallet 1992). In this context culturally appropriate services are defined as those services which emerge from Aboriginal communities and are consistent with the traditional cultures of Aboriginal people.

The adoption of the medicine wheel as a philosophical guide to service provision and the use of traditional practices in intervention, such as healing circles, sweat lodges and pipe ceremonies, have become more common (see Timpson et al. 1988; Longclaws 1994). As well, community-based holistic healing processes, such as that developed by Hollow Water First Nation (Lajeunesse 1993), have emerged as methods for intervention in neglect and abuse. While the incorporation of selected traditional practices contributes to the development of culturally appropriate services, a more comprehensive strategy is required. For example, McKenzie and Morrissette (1993) identify several factors which support the expansion of such services. These include recognition of: the importance of control over and provision of services by Aboriginal people; the effects of colonization and assimilation on Aboriginal people, and the need to provide services consistent with an individual's identification with Aboriginality; a distinct Aboriginal world view and the existence of traditional beliefs, values and customs which must be incorporated within models of helping; the role of elders, women and children in community life and the importance of building culturally appropriate services through community and staff participation; and the value of well managed organizations that strive to work with other informal and formal helping services toward more culturally appropriate interventions.

The process of policy analysis begins with an assessment of the problem, and in First Nations CFS this requires an understanding of the impact of culturally inappropriate models of service provision. This is most clearly illustrated by the historical pattern of removing Aboriginal children from their families and communities, and placing them in non-Aboriginal care, often on a permanent basis. These placement practices have begun to change, and joint placement planning for First Nations children is mandated by policy in Manitoba and elsewhere. Procedures which have been adopted give priority to out of home placement: first with the extended family; next with a community-based Aboriginal foster home; then with an Aboriginal resource outside the local community; and as a last resort with non-Aboriginal caregivers. These protocols have had a significant impact on placement practices, although cross-cultural placements still remain all too common. Two problems persist. First, some agencies make inadequate efforts to comply with these protocols. Second, there are not enough licensed Aboriginal caregivers to enable culturally appropriate placements for all Aboriginal children requiring out of home care. Culturally inappropriate services are also reflected in the limited attention to prevention, family preservation and family reunification. These policy issues have been of primary importance to West Region Child and Family Services and, while its service model has evolved over the past decade, there has been a consistent focus on the need to respond to these problems.

Case Study Results

The services and outcomes identified in this study were obtained during an evaluation of the programs of West Region CFS completed in 1994 (McKenzie 1994a), and involvement in an agency-sponsored participatory research project to develop First Nations CFS standards.

Agency Structure and Program Processes

The agency's service orientation is reflected in its statements of core values, major goals and philosophical beliefs. Core values stress the importance of protecting children within families and communities, the right to community self-determination and the importance of culture and traditions. Major goals express a commitment to prevention and support, the importance of repatriating children lost to member First Nations, efforts to retain children within their home community, and developing First Nations legislation and standards consistent with the goal of self-government. These purposes are summarized as four major philosophical principles which reflect the general value criteria to be used in assessing agency programs. These are: Aboriginal control; cultural relevancy; community-based services; and comprehensive, team oriented services.

The agency's philosophy and service model have been shaped by a number of factors but one of the most important is the socioeconomic context of its member communities. The communities served by the agency are characterized by a growing population and very high rates of unemployment and poverty. In addition, there is a limited service infrastructure, especially for specialized services related to sexual abuse, family violence, fetal alcohol syndrome and other special needs. These realities are connected to historical patterns of colonization that include residential schools and the separation of many First Nations children from their families by the conventional child welfare system.

Unlike many organizations, principles adopted by this agency are used both as guidelines for service planning and as criteria for assessing service quality. Principles of Aboriginal control and community-based services are reflected both in the agency's governance structures and service model. Decentralization is closely related to the concept "community-based," and three general models of consumerist oriented forms of social service decentralization have been identified (McKenzie 1994b). These are decentralized teams, community oriented decentralization and political decentralization. West Region CFS adheres to a model of political decentralization, that stresses community control and a collectivist approach to the sharing of power. The concept "community-based" is intended to describe the capacity of the local community to influence policy and service responses; thus, it is generally consistent with political decentralization. Local community involvement is reflected in the governance structure of West Region CFS. While the agency is separately incorporated outside the Tribal Council structure, it is governed by a board of Chiefs representing each of the First Nations served by the agency, and they espouse a strong commitment to agency goals, including community-based services, effectiveness and efficiency. Each community also has a local child and family service committee which meets regularly with community and supervisory staff on program development and case management issues.

The agency has adopted a service approach that includes locally-based staff and a focus on self-help and community building as well as the provision of individualized services. Community-based staff are the primary service providers and they are hired as either protection or prevention workers. They receive supervision and specialized service back-up from staff based at the regional office. However, supervisors and specialized staff from the child abuse, alternate (foster) care, treatment support and therapeutic foster care programs are assigned specific communities in order to promote a teamwork approach both with locally-based staff and community child and family service committees.

The abuse unit provides initial investigation services following referrals of abuse, and assists local workers who assume responsibility for follow-up services and case management. This model is quite effective in assuring required expertise in investigations, while protecting local community staff from some of the conflicts that can occur around initial abuse referrals in small communities. The treatment support unit was initially developed as an alternative to the purchase of costly clinical services from outside local communities, and the unit has expanded its staff complement in recent years. This unit is highly regarded because of its support to local staff and success in raising community consciousness about sexual abuse and other forms of family violence. The alternate care unit has primary responsibility for foster home recruitment, licensing and placement coordination. In 1994 there were about 190 foster homes, and approximately 90 of these were in use. The therapeutic foster care program has responsibility for training and support to foster parents providing care to children with special needs.

There are other efforts that promote a more community-based approach to service delivery. For example, a project to develop First Nations CFS standards within the region was based on a methodology that included two rounds of extensive community consultations. As well, the development of a new initiative to establish community-based intervention programs for sex offenders included a community consultation process in the planning phase. Of particular significance is the agency's efforts to involve community members in developing a strategic plan for the agency. Every two years a regional planning workshop is held and attended by a variety of community members from each First Nation. This serves two purposes: it provides an opportunity, in addition to the annual meeting, for accountability and feedback on current programs; and it serves as a basis for receiving community input on new service priorities. Results from this consultation, staff input and board direction are combined to produce a service development plan which serves as a strategic planning guide for the next two year cycle.

The cultural relevancy of services is shaped by individual and community identification with traditional values, but there is a consistent emphasis on the role of the extended family, the value of consensus building, and the involvement of elders. Three initiatives are important to highlight. The first is the importance attached to family, community and cultural connections. Permanency planning in the Aboriginal context implies a commitment to family continuity which is only now being proposed as a more general model in child welfare (McFadden and Downs 1995). Family continuity stresses practice first with the inner family circle, then with the extended family circle, and finally alternate placement with ongoing connections and links to the original family system. There is a strong adherence to placement policies which utilize extended family members as the option of first choice, and placement with Aboriginal resources within the child's own community as the next priority when out of home care is provided.

Cultural and community connections are important components of an Aboriginal approach to attachment theory. This has led to the development of an agency sponsored therapeutic foster home program which can be utilized as a culturally appropriate alternative to residential treatment or placement in treatment foster care within the conventional system. As well, family connections are stressed in all out of home placements, and the agency's efforts to facilitate family reunification occurs even in cases where permanent wardship has been granted.

A second initiative has involved the sponsorship of a community-based research project to compile First Nations CFS standards based on community and cultural preferences (see McKenzie, Seidl and Bone 1995).

Finally, the executive coordinator has designed an extensive supervisory training program based on the medicine wheel philosophy which was delivered to approximately half of the agency's staff members over an eighteen month period.

The commitment to comprehensive, team oriented services reflects a priority emerging from the limited range of service options available to communities, and the fact that previous patterns of utilizing outside professionals often led to intervention plans that failed to adequately consider the community and cultural context. These principles stress the importance of responding to children, families and communities within a holistic healing framework which makes use of a coordinated, multidisciplinary service response. A holistic context for healing is important because it transcends the notion of helping in the narrow therapeutic sense. Instead, it emphasizes the resilience of First Nations people, and their ability to utilize self-help and cultural traditions as a framework both for addressing problems and supporting future social development at the community level.

This approach to service delivery is reflected in staff expectations to work in partnership with others in the agency in order to respond to community needs. For example, local prevention and protection workers coordinate their service responses, and share responsibilities when required. Abuse and treatment support specialists participate in community outreach initiatives and provide consultation to community-based staff, as well as providing direct service. Two other policy initiatives embrace these principles. One is the direct sponsorship of a more comprehensive service response. For example, the agency sponsored a family violence initiative and developed child daycare programs in several communities. The treatment support unit has been instrumental in promoting community prevention and group programs, as well as providing individual and family counselling services. More recently, the agency has launched a community-based intervention program for sex offenders. A second initiative has involved a partnership arrangement with schools to develop school-based early intervention programs for youth.

There are several additional characteristics which are important. These are leadership and management functions, staff development and accountability. In most First Nations CFS agencies, high staff turnover, particularly among community-based staff, has been a persistent problem. In contrast, this agency has experienced a high rate of staff retention and a high level of staff morale. An important reason for this is the fact that senior management has provided consistent, supportive leadership that combines a progressive vision for service development with a practical focus on issues such as client oriented case management services and financial accountability. The latter issue deserves specific comment. Cost analysis and procedures related to financial accountability have been used by the agency to promote responsive planning and service development. For example, an analysis of the child maintenance fees for children with special needs, normally paid to other agencies for their care, was an important factor in the agency's decision to develop its own therapeutic foster care program. At the service delivery level, there has been a consistent emphasis on the provision of good quality supervision within a work environment where staff input and participation is highly valued. A high priority is placed on staff development, particularly for community-based staff without professional social work degrees. For example, the executive coordinator was a strong advocate of a distance education program in social work which is now being provided, and was directly involved in the provision of a supervisory training program for agency staff.

A key issue is that of resource adequacy. Most funding is provided by the federal government but funding policies are determined by the province, particularly in child maintenance. Agency management must negotiate and attempt to influence two levels of government both to obtain adequate levels of funding, and to secure sufficient flexibility for early intervention or new program initiatives. The relationship with provincial authorities has been most contentious in regard to funding. In general, the province has discouraged the development of new initiatives by its restrictive approaches to funding. For example, in 1993-94 it adopted a funding formula for children with special needs which did not provide adequate resources to respond to this group of children within West Region's catchment area. As well, it prohibits payments to biological families, a measure the agency utilizes, as required, to support family reunification. Recently, provincial authorities adopted a lower payment schedule for some extended family members providing foster family care. This unilaterally imposed policy is particularly discriminatory to First Nations agencies whose primary foster family resource is extended family members.

The agency's strategy in resource management has been threefold. It has adopted a strong advocacy stance with the federal and provincial levels of government to ensure some measure of adequacy. It has also stressed financial accountability and efficiency within its own operations, and reallocated resources as required to respond to new needs. As well, it was successful in negotiating a block funding agreement for child maintenance expenditures with the federal government in 1992. This allowed the agency to utilize funds, normally provided on a cost recovery basis for children in care, to provide a wider range of family support and treatment services. While surpluses may be carried forward, expenditures above the grant level are not recoverable unless exceptional circumstances exist. To date, this has not occurred and the new flexibility in funding afforded by this agreement has had a positive impact on program development.

Service Quality and Outcomes

In West Region, family support services are provided in an effort to maintain children within families. However, community outreach, particularly in relation to child sexual abuse and the identification of special needs, including fetal alcohol syndrome, have required a continuing emphasis on protection and child placement services. Family, community and cultural continuity reflect the basic mission of the child protection program but these are closely connected to a framework which incorporates family and community healing. Reunification, which is retained as an objective in most placements, depends both on effective placement planning and family-based intervention. The agency's placement protocols, affirmed by community members in the research project related to culturally appropriate standards, support reunification in that attachment with the extended family, community and culture is retained wherever possible. This policy is combined with a range of interventions provided to the family and the child by social workers, the treatment support team and other services. Successful reunifications are also facilitated by the ability to provide transitional financial support to the biological family if required.

Three approaches to the assessment of service quality were included in the evaluation. First, a provincial service audit of approximately one-half of the agency's files was conducted to examine service quality as indicated by file recording. The audit team concluded that there was a high degree of staff accountability for services, protection referrals were appropriately handled, and there was careful planning in relation to placements, including plans for family connections. Services were defined as above average and as having moved beyond basic protection to the provision of a range of support and treatment oriented interventions. Second, twelve intensive case studies were conducted utilizing information from file records and interviews with social workers. These demonstrated that a variety of efforts were being made to support family reunification through support services, counselling and other interventions. Finally, interviews with staff and a sample of foster parents were conducted. Staff described a shift in the agency's image over the past few years to a more supportive, community oriented approach to intervention. Community residents were described as more likely to utilize the agency as a source of help, and it was reported that voluntary requests for service had increased. Foster parents reported receiving more training and support services since the change in the agency's funding formula, and they expressed a high degree of satisfaction with agency services.

Trends pertaining to children in care are not always a reliable indicator of service effectiveness because a wide range of factors can affect these trends. However, they are more relevant when they are compared with trends elsewhere and considered in conjunction with an assessment of service quality. Between 1991 and 1994 the agency had a 4 percent decline in the number of children in care. While admissions to care in 1993-94 increased by 25 percent when compared with 1990-91, discharges from care were 45 percent higher in 1993-94. During this same period of time, the number of new admissions and the average number of children in care within the province increased significantly. An examination of "days in care" and expenditures for children in care confirms intake and discharge trends for West Region CFS. Between the fiscal year (FY) 91-92 and FY 93-94 the number of days in care provided by the agency declined by 4 percent and there was a 10 percent reduction in child maintenance costs. The two year comparison between FY 92-93 and FY 93-94 is perhaps more important because the impact of new programs, facilitated by the new funding agreement with the federal government, was not really apparent until FY 93-94. When this two year period is compared, the number of days care declined by 12 percent and there was a 10 percent reduction in child maintenance expenditures. Furthermore, it is important to note that these trends are not associated with any reduction in service quality, including the level of support services for families and children. Over the three year period the number of families and children served through support and treatment services increased significantly, and there was a 32 percent increase in expenditures to this program component alone.

An additional perspective on data related to children in care is provided by comparing trends for federally funded children in care in West Region CFS with those in other First Nations agencies. Between FY 91-92 and FY 93-94 the days in care for this group of children declined by 13 percent for West Region, whereas other agencies recorded an average increase of 9 percent. During the same period child maintenance costs declined by 19 percent for West Region whereas costs increased by an average of 11 percent in other First Nations agencies. Closer examination suggests that expenditure differences were related to two major factors: differences in trends for children in care and a higher reduction in the use of residential care in the case of West Region.

Placement trends were analyzed in detail to assess the stability of placement, compliance with agency policies on placement preferences and mobility. The evaluation also included a comparative analysis of placement practices both before and after the new funding formula. In the three years ending in 1993, slightly more than 80 percent of all placements involved foster family providers where there was at least one Aboriginal caregiver. More than one-half of all placements were made within the child's own community, and biological and extended family caregivers provided 42 percent of all days in care over this period of time. Moreover, placements with biological and extended family members increased when trends before and after the new funding formula were compared.

Placement stability is associated with success in out of home care, although some moves may be more disruptive than others. For example, some placements occur for relatively short periods of time, and other moves may be carefully planned to minimize disruption. Excluding successful family reunifications, 53 percent of all children in care had no moves over the three year period examined.

10 percent of children experienced four or more care providers, which might have included family members for periods of time. Permanent wards as a group had relatively stable placements, but there was a slight increase in mobility among all children when trends before and after the new funding formula were examined. This is a reflection of two factors. First, the agency was providing for more special needs children within its own resources, and placement stability is more difficult to achieve for some of these children. Second, the agency was placing an increased emphasis on family reunification, and not all of these placements resulted in continuing care within the biological family unit. Despite the modest increase in placement mobility, these results support the agency's general ability to achieve goals associated with family and cultural continuity.

A survey of outreach and community prevention programs was included to assess the implementation of group and community oriented services by prevention workers and staff with the treatment support unit between 1991 and 1994. Some of the more common continuing activities included support to child and family service committees, parent education programs, the organization of youth and summer camp programs, life skills programs and a regional men's group to deal with family violence. Significant efforts had been made to address issues related to sexual abuse, and a total of fifteen group programs for adolescents and adult women survivors had been sponsored. Other initiatives included cultural programs for youth, sharing circles, a youth drop-in centre and a program oriented to family empowerment.

The study also identified some issues that needed to be addressed in improving service quality. One example was the need to develop programs for sexual abuse offenders, an initiative which has now been established, and another involved efforts to strengthen the role of community child and family service committees. As well, recommendations were made for the extension of additional services related to victims of sexual abuse and children with fetal alcohol syndrome.

Perhaps the final reflection on agency programs should rest with community members, and data from participants at the 1994 regional planning workshop were analyzed as a indication of their views. Community respondents assigned a mean rating of 3.9 (where 1 = strongly disagree and 5 = strongly agree) in assessing the agency's general success in meeting its goals. Respondents were then asked to rank the two most important agency goals. These were to deliver community-based culturally appropriate services, and to attempt to keep children within their own community while ensuring that their best interests are met. As well, a high level of support was expressed for previous agency initiatives, including those related to treatment support, therapeutic foster care, family violence and the development of daycare services.

Conclusion

There are significant limitations in the ability of any child and family service program to reverse the effects of colonization on First Nations, particularly in relation to poverty and unemployment. Clearly, a strategy for economic development located within a sustainable development framework is required to realize social development goals in these communities. Furthermore, the principles and service model adopted by this agency may not be generalizable to other First Nations agencies because of differences in First Nations and agency leadership as well as community strengths and needs. There are also limitations to the variables addressed in this study, including the need for more attention to service outcomes. However, the study has demonstrated the general effectiveness of the agency's holistic approach to service delivery. It also illustrates that culturally appropriate practices in child protection can be combined with community prevention and outreach services over time to empower First Nations children, families and communities. Such a process is essential in establishing a basis for a self-government in First Nations which respects and values its most vulnerable members.

The framework used for this assessment focused on elements of a value analytic approach to policy analysis, system-level features such as leadership and staffing characteristics, and program evaluation criteria such as service quality, effectiveness and efficiency. The service model designed by the agency is based on four general principles which reflect the value criteria associated with the agency's mission. These are Aboriginal control, cultural relevancy, community-based services and a comprehensive, team oriented service response.

Several factors identified appeared to contribute to the agency's success. First, the agency has been able to achieve considerable autonomy and control over policies and services, as well as the ability to utilize much of its funding in more flexible and creative ways. This has required a considerable amount of advocacy with both levels of government because their standards and funding policies have had to be adapted to permit a more responsive and holistic service approach. In addition, the agency has been given appropriate autonomy by its board of Chiefs to manage its own budget and programs.

Second, agency leadership has combined a progressive vision for social development, sound program management skills that emphasize effectiveness and efficiency, and supportive staff development policies to create a working environment which is characterized by a high level of staff stability and commitment.

Finally, measures undertaken to reinforce community responsibility, involvement and accountability, including a participative approach to the development of standards, serve to reinforce a role for First Nations child and family services that transcends the old paradigm based on colonization and establishes one which is directed towards empowerment.

Note

1. The study on which this chapter is based was funded by the Department of Indian Affairs and Northern Development. Special appreciation is extended to agency staff who participated in the evaluation, Esther Seidl who reviewed a draft of the article, and Elsie Flette, the Executive Coordinator of West Region Child and Family Services, for her support in publishing these results.

Part 3:
Child and Family Poverty: Evaluating Income Support Programs and Policy Options

Campaign 2000:
Child and Family Poverty in Canada

DAVID I. HAY

Introduction

The United Nations designated 1996 as the International Year for the Eradication of Poverty. Many non-governmental organizations (NGOs) are pressuring governments to respond to this challenge by advancing public education activities on the issue of child and family poverty. These public education campaigns reveal the following facts about child and family poverty in Canada.[1]

• The latest available data (for 1994) point out that 1,362,000 children in Canada live in poverty,[2] which equals one out of every five children. This is an increase of 46 percent, or 428,000 children, since 1989 (Campaign 2000 1996b).
• Child poverty has risen because the value of income supports have declined: median family income has decreased $5,000 since 1989; the value of the federal child tax benefit is decreasing; and social assistance rates are generally lower (BC Campaign 2000 1996a).
• Child poverty has also risen because it is increasingly difficult to achieve income security through employment. The number of children in families experiencing long term unemployment has increased over 50 percent since 1989. Although there has been a net increase in jobs created since 1989, there has been a decrease in full-time jobs. Many of the new jobs created are part-time, at lower wages and without benefits. As a result, the number of children in working poor families has increased 37 percent since 1989 (Campaign 2000 1995b).

The *United Nations Human Development Reports* (United Nations Development Program 1990, 1991, 1992, 1994, 1995) consistently rank Canada at or near the top of all countries in human development, and this is widely quoted by government officials. Canada's ranking drops noticeably in these reports when the number of children living in poverty is included. Canada's rate of child poverty is worse than all other major Western countries, with the exception of Australia and the United States (Hay 1993a).

Overall, the intentions of this chapter are to provide an overview of some of the "behind-the-scenes" issues involved in child and family poverty and to promote more informed debate about potential solutions.[3] Specifically, the chapter describes the activities of Campaign 2000, one of the organizations working to end child and family poverty in Canada. As well, the dimensions and consequences of child and family poverty and the policy mechanisms used or proposed to alleviate poverty are considered. Also included in this chapter is an examination of the distribution and trends in income security for Canadians. The chapter concludes with a discussion of the prospects for developments that will begin to reverse the rising trend in child and family poverty, working towards its eradication by the year 2000.

What is Campaign 2000?

Campaign 2000 is a national social movement that aims to build awareness and support for programs and policies to end child poverty in Canada. Campaign 2000 is a non-partisan coalition of eighteen national partners and a network of thirty-one provincial and community partner organizations in every Canadian province. Partners represent just about every interest in the not-for-profit sector including: anti-poverty, children's groups, housing, food banks, faith, social planning, health and immigrant women.[4] Through advocacy, political lobbying, media events, partnership with a major retail business and numerous public education activities, Campaign 2000 has given a national profile to the issue of child poverty (Popham, Hay and Hughes forthcoming).

On November 24, 1989, after years of education and lobbying by groups such as the Child Poverty Action Group, the Canadian Council on Social Development and the Canadian Council on Children and Youth, a resolution was passed unanimously in the House of Commons of Canada: "to seek to achieve the goal of eliminating poverty among Canadian children by the year 2000" (Canada House of Commons 1989). Representatives of the three official parties spoke passionately to the resolution, moved by Ed Broadbent (Leader of the New Democratic Party), seconded by Jean Charest (Minister of Youth, Progressive Conservative Party) and defended by Lloyd Axworthy (Liberal Party Member of Parliament).

To hold Canadian politicians accountable to their commitment, on November 24, 1991, Campaign 2000 was publicly launched with the declaration, "we are committed to promoting and securing the full implementation of the House of Commons Resolution of November 24, 1989" (Campaign 2000 1992:n.p.). Since the fall of 1991, national and provincial partner organizations and others involved with Campaign 2000 have conducted political lobbying and public education activities to keep the issue of child poverty high on the public and political agenda (G. York 1991). For example, Campaign 2000:

> • presents briefs to federal government committees, commissions and task forces;
> • corresponds and holds meetings with all members of Parliament and key provincial ministers on an ongoing basis to remind them of their commitment to do something about child and family poverty and to

discuss potential solutions;
• actively organizes, supports and delivers many public education events on child and family poverty;
• with its community partners and others, identifies and takes action on poverty issues in their communities.

Beginning in 1992, Campaign 2000 has produced annual *Child Poverty in Canada* report cards to monitor the changing conditions of families and children (Campaign 2000 1992, 1993, 1994b, 1995b, 1996b). Community partners have also produced annual report cards (see for example, BC Campaign 2000 1995, 1996b, 1996c, 1996d, Metro Campaign 2000 1995). Generally, Campaign 2000 members release their report cards publicly at news conferences in November of each year, on or near the anniversary date of the House of Commons resolution.

Since 1991, BC Campaign 2000 has been an active coalition of community groups working together to promote public education and political action on child poverty issues in BC.[5] This year, in addition to producing our second annual report card, *Child Poverty in BC: Report Card 1996* (BC Campaign 2000 1996b), BC Campaign 2000 developed and produced a *Child Poverty Community Action Kit* to provide others throughout BC with information, ideas and tools to take action on child poverty issues (BC Campaign 2000 1996a). On November 18, 1996 (the public release date for the national and BC report cards in 1996), a number of news conferences and other activities took place in Vancouver and at least twelve other BC communities acknowledging the seriousness of child and family poverty.[6]

Child and Family Poverty in Canada: Dimensions, Effects and Consequences

Canadian Dimensions

In the spring of 1996, the Canadian Council on Social Development published a detailed chartbook on child and family poverty (Ross, Scott and Kelly 1996). The opening chart in this publication makes it clear that the extent of child and family poverty very much depends on family type (the chart is reproduced here as Figure 1).[7] In 1993, among all families in Canada, 1.1 million—15 percent of Canadian families—were deemed to be poor. The poverty rate goes as high as 81 percent, however, for never-married female single parents whose children are under seven years of age.

Poverty rates also vary by place of residence. Based on data from the 1991 census, Lochhead and Shillington (1996) found that poverty rates for Canada's twenty-five largest urban areas ranged from a high of 22 percent in Montreal, to a low of 9 percent in Oshawa, Ontario. Four of the top seven cities were in Quebec (Montreal, Trois-Rivières, Sherbrooke and Quebec City).

As well, poverty rates can vary enormously depending on where within a

Figure 1
Poverty Rates Among Canadian Families, 1993

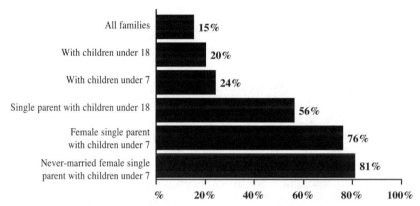

* Poverty is measured using Statistics Canada's Low Income Cut-offs (LICOS). 1986 base (for the years 1981 to 1991) and 1992 base (for 1992 to 1994).

Source: Prepared by the Centre for International Statistics at the CCSD, using Statistics Canada's Survey of Consumer Finances microdata tape.

Figure 2
Child Poverty Rate in Canada, Selected Years

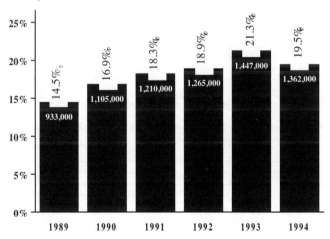

* Poverty is measured using Statistics Canada's Low Income Cut-offs (LICOS). 1986 base (for the years 1981 to 1991) and 1992 base (for 1992 to 1994).

Source: Prepared by the Centre for International Statistics at the CCSD, based on Statistics Canada's *Income Distributions by Size in Canada, 1991, 1993* and *1994*.

particular city a person lives. For example, when poverty rates in Vancouver were examined by census local areas, the rates ranged from a low of 8 percent in West Point Grey and Dunbar-Southlands to a high of over 50 percent in Mount Pleasant (54 percent) and Strathcona (52 percent) (City of Vancouver 1994, 1991 census data).

Ross, Scott and Kelly (1996:4) remark that "child poverty is a persistent problem in Canada." This was recently acknowledged in a Human Resources Development Canada research paper entitled "Why Has the Child Poverty Rate Failed to Fall?" (Human Resources Development Canada 1996b; Zyblock 1996a). Similarly, in a paper examining low income among Canadian children, Picot and Myles (1995) report that the proportion of children in low-income families has been "relatively stable" from 1973 to 1991.[8]

Figure 2 shows the Canadian child poverty rate for the years 1989 to 1994. Poverty rates show similar trends within each Canadian province, although percentages for 1994 range from a low of 13 percent in Prince Edward Island to nearly 24 percent in Newfoundland (National Council of Welfare 1996). British Columbia's child poverty rate was below the national average in 1989 at 13.6 percent, but BC's 1994 rate of 19.9 percent was above the Canadian average (BC Campaign 2000 1996c; National Council of Welfare 1996).[9]

Table 1a and 1b
Percentage Distributions of Families with Children by Relative Income Category.[1] Gross Income

Table 1a. All Families with Children						
Percent who	Australia	Canada	Germany	Sweden	United Kingdom	United States
Are Poor	18.59	17.67	8.82	4.71	16.63	25.41
Are Near Poor	7.41	8.28	9.28	6.87	10.11	8.23
Are in the Middle	56.89	57.82	67.69	79.29	52.85	48.56
Are Affluent	17.12	16.23	14.20	9.03	20.41	17.81

Table 1b. Single-Parent Families						
Percent who	Australia	Canada	Germany	Sweden	United Kingdom	United States
Are Poor	53.19	48.83	32.09	8.29	25.00	53.92
Are Near Poor	7.80	8.74	13.98	12.15	25.23	7.26
Are in the Middle	30.85	36.46	49.21	75.69	40.97	32.11
Are Affluent	7.80	6.18	4.92	3.31	8.80	6.71

1. Families are defined as "poor" if equivalent gross income is less than 50 percent of median equivalent gross income for the country; for "near-poor" with 50-62.5 percent of median equivalent gross income, middle-class with 62.5-1.5 times median equivalent gross income and with more than 1.5 times median equivalent income. Equivalent gross income is calculated as family gross income divided by the OECD scale.

Source: Phipps 1993.

International Dimensions

A number of recent publications provide information that contrasts Canada's poverty rates with selected Organization for Economic Cooperation and Development (OECD) countries (Baker 1995a; Phipps 1993, 1996; Ross, Shillington and Lochhead 1994).

Tables 1a and 1b present comparative information for Canada and five other OECD countries on the percentage distribution of families by income group. Using 1987 data from the Luxembourg Income Study, Table 1a shows that nearly 18 percent of Canadian families with children were poor.[10] This is better than Australia and the United States, but much worse than Sweden and Germany. Similarly, Table 1b shows that "single-parent families are at much greater risk [of poverty] in Canada than in many other countries" (Phipps 1993:3).

Poverty's Effects and Consequences

Common sense and numerous research studies point to the conclusion that lack of income hampers healthy child development. For example, a 1996 food costing survey shows that families living in poverty cannot afford to meet the nutritional needs of their children (BC Campaign 2000 1996d; Yeung 1996). The average cost of a nutritious food basket for a family of four is $741.66 per month (Yeung 1996). A family of four in BC living on social assistance receives $589 per month for *all* support costs (Province of British Columbia. Ministry of Social Services 1996c).[11] The medical health officer for the Capital Regional District (i.e., Victoria, BC and greater metropolitan area) has stated that "nutrition and food security are the cornerstones in achieving the Health Goals for both the region and the province . . . [p]overty is at the root of many health problems, including being a barrier to nutritious food" (Yeung 1996:5).

Poverty is recognized as the single most significant indicator of health status (*Globe and Mail* 1996a; Hay 1994). The health problems of poor children begin before birth and continue to place these children at greater risk of death, disability and other health problems throughout their lives (Epp 1986; Federal, Provincial and Territorial Advisory Committee on Population Health 1994, 1996; Hay 1994; Rivers 1996; Scott 1996b; Yeung 1996). Health problems of poor kids frequently become chronic as adults, and by that time increasing income has much less effect on health (Hay 1993b).

Poor children are twice as likely to have their school performance judged as "poor" by their teachers, more likely to miss school and twice as likely to drop out before graduating. Not completing school means less chance of finding work (Ross, Scott and Kelly 1996). Poor children are also more likely to be hyperactive; suffer from emotional disorders; exhibit disorderly conduct; get into trouble with the law; be in the care of child welfare services; engage in riskier behaviours (smoking, drinking and taking drugs); and be unemployed as adults (Scott 1996b).

What is the experience of poverty for the poor? Living in poverty means children are not able to live up to their potential. Growing up poor hurts children: they are derided for the way they look, the way they talk, where they live and so on. Poverty has devastating effects on the self-esteem of poor children and their families (Baxter 1993; Judy Swanson 1996; Toupin 1994). Increasingly the poor are being blamed for their own poverty when substantial evidence points to the lack of job opportunities and adequate social supports as the reason that people are living in poverty (First Call 1996).

Child poverty has implications for all Canadians. Children are the future workforce, the parents of the next generation and the support for an aging population. Canada's high standard of living cannot be developed and maintained by an increasingly poor, unhealthy and vulnerable population of children.

Family Income: Sources, Adequacy and Inequality

Income Sources

Families receive the majority of their income through the employment earnings of one or more family members. However, most families receive income from sources other than employment earnings. Savings, investments and government program transfers (cash and tax credits) are examples of these other income sources. Tax and transfer income (e.g., Canada pension plan, old age security, guaranteed income supplement, employment insurance, child tax benefit, GST tax credit, RRSP deductions, childcare expense deduction and so on) are more or less important depending on family income level.

Table 2 shows that the 20 percent of Canadian families with the lowest incomes had an average "market" income (wages, salaries, interest and dividends before direct government transfers) of $925 in 1993. These Canadian families relied on an average of $9,148 in government transfers, 91 percent of their income. In comparison, the top 20 percent of Canadian families received on average $1,493 in direct transfers, less than 2 percent of their average total income of $93,207 (from market income and transfers).

Table 2

Average Pre-tax Market Income (employment, savings and investments) and Government Income Transfers (cash and tax credits) by Quintile for Canadian families (1991 constant dollars)

FAMILIES	1973		1993	
	Market	Transfer	Market	Transfer
Bottom 20%	$1,961 (27%)	$5,269 (73%)	$925 (9%)	$9,148 (91%)
Fourth 20%	$16,618 (83%)	$3,486 (17%)	$13,773 (64%)	$7,836 (36%)
Middle 20%	$30,888 (93%)	$2,209 (7%)	$30,519 (87%)	$4,438 (13%)
Second 20%	$45,250 (96%)	$1,921 (4%)	$49,485 (94%)	$3,093 (6%)
Top 20%	$78,233 (98%)	$1,796 (2%)	$91,714 (98%)	$1,493 (2%)

Source: Compiled from Sharpe 1996:1–2.

Many families in the poorest 20 percent include people not in the labour force, some who are unable to participate (i.e., seniors, disabled, students, "potential"[12] workers and others). Thus, government transfers are very important, especially for the poor.

Picot and Myles (1995, 1996) report that the "relative stability" in the number of children in low income families over the period 1973 to 1991 was achieved through a combination of changing family structure, decreasing employment earnings and increasing transfer payments. Given the changes in the labour market and government income transfer programs, it is important to examine the consequences of current trends in these income sources, particularly from 1992 (Battle 1995; Little 1996; Sharpe 1996).

What's Happening to Family Income?

Employment

The labour market is in transition. This means that full-time, adequately paying and secure jobs are disappearing. Jobs created tend to be part-time, lower paying and less secure (Social Planning and Research Council of BC 1996). Child poverty rates rise and fall with unemployment rates (Novick and Shillington 1996). In 1994, 457,000 full-time jobs were created and the national child poverty rate fell nearly 2 percentage points from the previous year (Campaign 2000 1996b). Almost all of the 88,000 jobs gained in 1995 were part-time (Ecumenical Coalition for Economic Justice 1996). The effect of this much more modest job increase on child poverty rates remains to be seen.[13]

Minimum wages are inadequate to keep most people out of poverty. A family of four with one person working full-time at the BC minimum wage ($7 per hour, the highest in Canada) would be approximately $17,000 *below* the poverty line (BC Campaign 2000 1996b). As well, the distribution of employment income is increasingly unequal (Battle 1995; Human Resources Development Canada 1996c; Little 1996; Sharpe 1996; Zyblock 1996b). "In 1992, upper-

Table 3
Big Profits and Big Job Losses (1995 data)

Company	Profits (millions)	Jobs Lost
General Motors	1,391	2,500
Bell Canada	502	3,170
CIBC	1,015	1,289
Bank of Montreal	986	1,428
Petro Canada	196	564
Maritime Tel	32	471
Shell Canada	523	471

Source: Ecumenical Coalition for Economic Justice 1996:9.

income families' slice of the market income pie was twenty-two times larger than that of low-income families — the widest gap since Statistics Canada began calculating incomes, as of 1981" (Battle 1995:5). In part, this reflects the "jobless growth" of the new economy where companies reporting record profits continue to reduce the number of their employees (see Table 3). While public sector job reductions are usually the result of spending cuts for purposes of deficit reduction, private sector jobs tend to be lost because of "the passionate pursuit of productivity and competitiveness that pervades Canada's economy" (Ip 1996:D1).

Income Transfer Programs
Despite declining market income for the bottom three quintiles (Table 2) and growth in contingent casualized forms of employment, federal and provincial governments are reducing the level of assistance available through income transfer programs. Consider the following examples. Fewer and fewer workers are able to receive employment insurance benefits if they lose their job. For those workers who are able to collect benefits, the amount of the benefit and the number of weeks you can collect it continue to be reduced (Pulkingham and Ternowetsky 1997). In many Canadian provinces social assistance benefits have been reduced, eligibility has been restricted and marginal tax rates for recipients earning employment income are 75 percent in provinces such as BC (Province of British Columbia 1995).

Some people advocate cutting benefits and restricting program eligibility for government income transfer programs even further (BC Campaign 2000 1996c; Ekos Research Associates 1995; Biggs 1996). Higher income Canadians (who are less reliant on transfers) are the ones in favour of cutting government spending on programs, while other Canadians, generally speaking, are not (Ekos Research Associates 1995; Biggs 1996).

Given an "uncertain" labour market and a decreasing program role for governments, more and more families are feeling economically insecure (Ip 1996). In summary, the evidence seems to indicate that both jobs with adequate wages and benefits *and* strong government income transfer programs are needed to reduce poverty and ensure income security for Canadians.[14]

Child and Family Income Policies

Policy Environment
Over the years governments have introduced a number of child and family income policies (Baker 1995a, 1994; Hess 1992, 1993; Human Resources Development Canada 1994b; Ross 1983). As the preceding section has shown, however, federal and provincial income transfer programs are being cut back. The arguments from governments are that current levels of spending for income transfer programs are not affordable as they contribute to annual budgetary deficits and accumulated government debts (Hay 1995a; Novick and Shillington

1996; Pulkingham and Ternowetsky 1996b). A widely quoted study by Statistics Canada economists Mimoto and Cross (1991), however, found that 94 percent of the amount of the federal debt can be attributed to foregone revenue in the form of reduced taxes on corporations and higher income individuals, and rising expenditures in the form of interest payments on the debt. Furthermore 6 percent of the debt can be attributed to *all* program spending (Hay 1995a; Mimoto and Cross 1991; Pulkingham and Ternowetsky 1996b). Mendelson (1995) has convincingly shown that spending cuts alone will not get rid of the debt. In fact, the size of the federal debt will continue to grow even with no year-to-year budgetary deficits. Unless something is done to increase revenues, maintain low real interest rates *and* make spending cuts, "doing the math" shows that Canada will continue to pay an ever increasing portion of federal revenues towards paying down the debt (Mendelson 1995).

One of the ways that federal social program expenditures were reduced was in a policy implemented on April 1, 1996. This was the date that marked the end of the Canada Assistance Plan (CAP), and the beginning of the Canada Health and Social Transfer (CHST) (Pulkingham and Ternowetsky 1996b). The CAP had an important principle that the CHST does not: a legislated commitment by governments to provide financial assistance to anyone in need, whatever the cause of that need (Hess 1992, 1993; Human Resources Development Canada 1994b). Provincial governments were free to interpret what level of financial assistance they felt to be adequate, but they had to provide something to any person who could demonstrate need. This small protection has been lost with the introduction of the Canada Health and Social Transfer. Provinces are now free to provide assistance only to whomever *they* deem to be deserving.[15]

Earlier it was shown that Canada has one of the highest child poverty rates of all OECD countries. It was also implied that increased public spending may be necessary to reduce (let alone eradicate) child and family poverty in Canada. Given the Canadian fiscal context for the development of income transfer policies, it is interesting to contrast Canada's public expenditures on income security with other countries (Baker 1995a; Novick and Shillington 1996; Phipps 1993, 1995a, 1995b, 1996). Canada spends less (12 percent) than the OECD average (17 percent) for income security programs (Campaign 2000 1993, 1994b, 1995b). "In a study of twenty countries, Canada ranked sixteenth in income security spending as a percentage of GDP [gross domestic product]" (Campaign 2000 1994b:n.p.). As well, "Canada provides the least generous basic child benefit to median income families among major industrialized countries" (Novick and Shillington 1996:15). Predictably, countries with the lowest spending have the highest child poverty rates (Campaign 2000 1995b). Further, although Canadians complain that combined levels of taxation are already too high and hence cannot be increased (Shillington 1996), Canada's total tax revenue as a percentage of GDP (1992 data) is below the OECD average (Campaign 2000 1994b).

BC Benefits: A program example

The BC government recently changed its social assistance legislation to create BC Benefits (Province of British Columbia 1995). BC Benefits provide income and other supports for low income people. The BC government says BC Benefits are "Canada's most balanced and progressive set of social programs" (Province of British Columbia 1995:8). Indeed there are some positive features of BC Benefits, specifically the Healthy Kids and Family Bonus programs.

Healthy Kids is a program that provides dental and vision care benefits for children in low income working families (with no other available coverage). The lack of extended health benefit coverage for some low income working families has been cited as a potential barrier in moving off social assistance and into the labour force (Province of British Columbia 1995). The Family Bonus program is "a significant new financial benefit for low and modest income families . . . [and] a tangible action to address family poverty" (Province of British Columbia 1995:10). The Family Bonus provides a monthly cheque of $103 per child per month to working families with children. The amount of the benefit is reduced as family income increases. For example, families receive maximum benefits at $18,000 of family net income, while a family with two children would no longer receive benefits once their net income was above $32,000 (Province of British Columbia 1995:10).[16]

Some of the changes introduced with BC Benefits were not as positive, however (BC Campaign 2000 1996b; End Legislated Poverty 1996). Singles and couples without children had their support allowances cut back ($46 or 20 percent for singles, $92 or 10 percent for couples) (Province of British Columbia 1996c). This leaves singles with $325 a month for housing and $175 (less than $6 per day) for all other expenses, including food (see Figure 3 for a comparison between amounts provided to people receiving BC Benefits and the poverty line). The earnings exemption has been eliminated. 75 percent of all earned income is kept by the government. Previously, families were able to keep the first $200 of employment earnings, singles could keep the first $100, and both could keep 25 percent of earnings above this amount (BC Campaign 2000

Figure 3:
Adequacy of BC Social Assistance Benefits

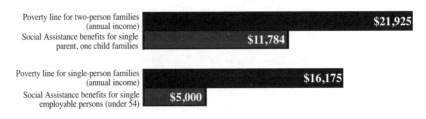

Poverty line for two-person families (annual income) — $21,925
Social Assistance benefits for single parent, one child families — $11,784

Poverty line for single-person families (annual income) — $16,175
Social Assistance benefits for single employable persons (under 54) — $5,000

Source: BC Campaign 2000 1996b.

1996b). Another change introduced with BC Benefits means that assistance is denied to people without children who have not lived in BC for at least three months. This change means that recent migrants to BC who lose their jobs and are not eligible for employment insurance will have no other public means to obtain financial support. With the introduction of the Youth Works program, the Province of British Columbia (1996c:12) maintains that it is "ending welfare for young people" by providing support to 19-24 year olds "if they participate in job search and work preparation programs." However, Youth Works programs (e.g., career planning, skills plan development, job-finding clubs, training and work experience) are only available to youth who receive benefits continuously for seven months or longer (Province of British Columbia 1996c). A majority of youth leave BC Benefits after three months (BC Campaign 2000 1996b).

The following story provides an illustration of what some of these changes may mean to BC Benefits recipients (BC Campaign 2000 1996b:n.p.). Beth is a single mother with an 8 year old son named John. They both live on an income assistance cheque of $982 per month. Prior to the introduction of BC Benefits, Beth relied on various part-time jobs to supplement her assistance and usually was able to earn around $500, $275 of which she and John were able to keep. The money helped to pay Beth's employment related expenses (clothes, transportation and childcare), and the jobs helped Beth remain active in the workforce and make contacts for more secure employment. The changes introduced by BC Benefits means that now Beth can only keep $125 of her employment earnings. Unfortunately, this is not enough to cover her expenses, and Beth is wondering how she can be worse off financially after working.

Policy Goals and Values
The goal of ending child and family poverty will be easily achieved by providing all Canadians with an adequate income. The means to achieve this goal are much more difficult and complex however, and what are deemed to be appropriate policy options depends to a great extent on the underlying assumptions and values of politicians, policy makers and the public at large. It is important to review these underlying assumptions and values to help guide policy choices.

In recent years a number of reports have examined Canadian values (Peters 1995) and proposed "frameworks" and "paradigms" of well-being (Rioux and Hay 1993; Roeher Institute 1993) as new approaches to understanding social welfare. Traditionally, approaches to understanding well-being have assumed that everyone is similar to everyone else, and that well-being can be measured and ranked according to a universal list of individual needs, usually economic ones (Doyal and Gough 1991; Drover and Kerans 1993). Alternatively, these new approaches define well-being as a dynamic process in which people are seen as linked together in ever widening circles of interpersonal and institutional interrelatedness, grounded in genuine concern for the well-being of others, feelings about what is fair and what people should be able to expect from one another (Rioux and Hay 1993). These links are nurtured by attitudes of mutual respect: people are valued for no particular reason except the fact that they are human and involved in the same human condition. Such ties humanize what would otherwise be purely a society of self-seeking individuals engaged in mutual exploitation for their own purposes (Rioux and Hay 1993).

Definitions of well-being highlight the ever present tension between individual (or group) choices and interdependence. This tension is very evident in discussions of policy options to deal with child and family poverty (Allen 1995; Eichler 1988c; Kitchen 1994; McDaniel 1990; Newman 1996; O'Neill 1994; Phipps 1995b; Valpy 1993). Phipps (1995b:187) explicitly states her orientation to assessing "tax and transfer options" for child and family income security as being that "the principle goal for our child-related policies should be increased equality in the distribution of well-being among Canadian children—with reasonably high standards for all."[17] In an article that comments directly on Phipps (1995b), Allen takes the opposite viewpoint, arguing that Phipps is "misguided," and that the "egalitarian bias of [Phipps'] paper needs a reality check from first economic principles" (1995:274). However, as Allen himself admits, "economic theory is quite useless in articulating exactly what people want and how it should be provided" (1995:274).[18]

The field of economics, as Allen (1995) helpfully reminds us, is without its own set of (explicit) values. The biggest failure of the private market is in the distribution of resources (generally money) to adequately meet the daily living requirements of citizens. And while it is increasingly difficult to think of public policy in anything other than economic terms, social policy is more traditionally defined as the deliberate intervention by government, and other sectors in society,[19] to address human requirements that are not adequately provided for, or distributed by, the private market (Hess 1993). As such, social policy is explicitly value driven. And as more people are realizing that policy decisions should not be made in separate realms because social, economic and fiscal policy are interrelated and interdependent (Rioux and Hay 1993), at some point economists will also have to embrace and explicitly incorporate value positions into their work (Caledon Institute of Social Policy 1996; Scott 1996b).[20]

Policy Options

On November 18, 1996, Campaign 2000 released *Crossroads for Canada: A Time to Invest in Children and Families* (Novick and Shillington 1996). This paper builds on Campaign 2000's 1994 policy discussion paper (1994c) that proposed a "life cycle strategy for healthy child development" (Novick and Shillington 1996:2). The premise of the *Crossroads for Canada* paper is that social investments in children and families have to be made a national priority and that new approaches to investments are needed. The paper argues that two to two-and-one-half percent of GDP should be redirected to a social investment strategy with the following five objectives:

128

• create a floor of decent living standards for modest and low income families;

• endow all young children with the stimulation and care for a healthy start in life;

• provide parents with family-time options during formative periods of their children's lives;

• protect the living standards of children when parental separation occurs; and

• assure every academically qualified child in Canada financial access to post-secondary training and studies, without having to incur massive debts into adulthood. (Novick and Shillington 1996:5)

There are three major components of the proposed social investment fund (Novick and Shillington 1996:28-36). The first is a comprehensive child benefit system with three sub-components: an enhanced basic child benefit—at its maximum value ($4,200 per child), it would be approximately four times the current federal child tax benefit ($1,020 per child); a family care supplement to "top-up the basic child benefit to the poverty line for lone parents and couples on limited earnings" (Novick and Shillington 1996:31); and an advanced maintenance payment system for child support to maintain the living standards of parents in receipt of child support. The second is a "national envelope for provinces to develop a comprehensive early development and child care system in every community across Canada" (Novick and Shillington 1996:28). The proposal would designate a "benchmark" proportion of GDP (e.g., 0.5–1 per-cent) to the envelope and develop a plan to achieve it. The third is a national youth education endowment plan, whereby a "public endowment of up to $20,000" (Novick and Shillington 1996:28) would be set aside for educational support. Access to the endowment would be family income tested, as would be the total amount available for support.

Specific policy mechanisms for the delivery of the social investment fund components remain to be developed, but they would be judged against the fund's objectives and the "five critical dimensions of well-being" outlined in the paper (Novick and Shillington 1996:7-10).[21]

The Novick and Shillington (1996:33) paper also addresses how Canadians would finance the social investment fund proposal, a fund "that when fully implemented would require . . . $16–$20 billion in new public revenue." Recognizing "the culture of tax resistance in Canada," the authors propose three areas to be tapped for revenue: government would preserve current expenditure levels in areas covered by the fund; a designated "special tax" on gross income would be implemented and is estimated to raise $5 billion; and special corporate capital taxes "with appropriate exemptions for small business" would be introduced (Novick and Shillington 1996:35-36).

It remains to be seen what the reaction to the social investment fund proposal will be from government and the policy making community. Media response has been less than favourable, however. *The Vancouver Sun* (1996a:A13) ran a feature article that outlined the characteristics of the fund, and the headline asked, "Child Poverty: Is the Solution More Taxes?" An editorial the next day answered that question with its headline "Work, Not Taxes" (*Vancouver Sun* 1996b:A14), and argued that job creation, not an "aggressive program of income redistribution . . . is the only solution to the problem of child poverty." The editor-in-chief of *The Globe and Mail* (Thorsell 1996:D8) side-stepped the policy debates and proposed that education and training of low income parents in appropriate values and childrearing practices would help children in poverty by going "to the root of the problem."

At the same time as policy advocacy groups such as Campaign 2000 are proposing their policy solutions to alleviate child and family poverty, the "hottest" policy talk for children and families is of a federal–provincial initiative to deliver a comprehensive national child benefit (Gadd 1996b; *Globe and Mail* 1996b, 1996c, 1996d; Greenspon 1996a, 1996b, 1996c). Currently no specifics on what federal and provincial ministers are discussing have been made public. All that has been shared is that a national child benefit will most likely consist of a "roll-up" of the federal child tax benefit with provincial monies currently given to low income families with children (primarily social assistance payments) (Greenspon 1996c). The benefit would be administered by the federal government in cooperation with provincial governments. Overall, this proposal may be similar to the BC Benefits Family Bonus discussed earlier in this chapter. The cost of such a benefit is rumoured in media reports to require an additional $1–$2 billion. How the benefit will be financed (i.e., through a redistribution of current program spending or through increased revenues) is unknown. January 1997 has been given as a timeline for the completion of a national child benefit proposal (Greenspon 1996c).

It is beyond the scope of this chapter to begin a discussion of the multitude of child and family benefit alternatives. A number of authors provide comprehensive reviews of policy goals, issues and options (Battle and Muszynski 1995; Gadd 1996a; Kesselman 1994; Mendelson 1996; Naylor 1995; Phipps 1995a; Woolley, Vermaeten and Madill 1996).[22] Of note, Phipps (1995a) concludes that a universal child allowance, paid monthly, should replace the child tax benefit and earned income supplement. Phipps (1995a:211-12) reasons that "universal cash transfers are preferable to tax exemptions or credits in at least five important ways:"[23] they are administratively efficient (no calculations to determine eligibility are required); they are automatically available to help families experiencing sudden reductions in income, an experience which is increasingly common in today's labour market; they do not generate negative work incentives since they are available regardless of parents' labour market attachment; countries with generous universal child benefits have much lower rates of child poverty than does Canada; and evidence from other countries suggest that generous universal benefits are popular, helping to ensure that their value will not erode during difficult economic times. This is particularly important from the perspective of children in low income families. In a policy environment characterized primarily by proposals to increase the targeting of income transfer programs, the proposal put forth by Phipps (1995a) stands out.

Conclusion

Canadians like to think of themselves as members of a caring and compassionate community (Peters 1995). One way that we can see evidence of these values in Canadian society is in the public support systems that have been put in place: social services, health care, minimum wages and employment standards, income support programs (social assistance, pensions, employment insurance) and so on. In the last number of years, however, we have started to experience a move away from values of community and towards values of individual choice (Valpy 1993).

This shift may be understandable in the context of increasing insecurity for many Canadian families and when "we can't afford it" and "there is no alternative" become public mantras. All indications are, however, that this shift will produce greater security for a few Canadians, and less security for most. Concurrently with this shift in values has come a shift in support for publicly delivered community support services. In times of fiscal difficulty, it seems that the money for these services are first, and most heavily, cut. The short term effect of program spending cuts will mean that budgets *may* be balanced sooner than later. It is clear, however, that the long term effects of these policy choices may be severe, leading to increased social and economic inequality, which has the potential of increasing costs for governments as more people will need to use health care, income support programs, victims services and so on. Deficits and debts are important issues, but deficits and debts should not be so important that people, communities and values get short shrift.

This chapter began by noting that 1996 was the United Nations International Year for the Eradication of Poverty. The United Nations also announced that the International Year 1996 would be followed by a Decade for the Eradication of Poverty. It is hoped that the will of politicians and the public may unite to promote action to end child and family poverty by the year 2000.

Political *and* public will is needed to begin the work towards ending child poverty in Canada. Politicians must have plans and policies to help create jobs; to ensure adequate incomes; to support childcare; and to ensure that secure, adequate and affordable housing is available for all. But, the public has to make politicians, and other people in our community, aware that Canada's child and family poverty is an international disgrace.

Notes

1 . See the following references for information on the dimensions and consequences of child and family poverty: BC Campaign 2000 1995, 1996a,1996b; Campaign 2000 1992, 1993, 1994b, 1995b, 1996b; Ross, Scott and Kelly 1996; Ross, Shillington and Lochhead 1994; Scott 1996b.

2 . Throughout this chapter poverty is measured using Statistics Canada Low Income Cut-offs (LICOs) unless otherwise noted.

3 . Although given the current level of public activity in this area, how long a reader may be informed by this chapter's content is an open question.

4 . For a fuller discussion of the development of Campaign 2000, particularly as a social movement, see Popham, Hay and Hughes forthcoming.

5 . The Social Planning and Research Council (SPARC) of BC, First Call!!–BC Child and Youth Advocacy Coalition, the BC Teachers' Federation and others are currently active members in BC Campaign 2000.

6 . For a listing of communities, their activities and local contacts, see BC Campaign 2000 1996c. The BC Campaign 2000 news conference had wide coverage in the BC print, radio and television media. For newspaper reports on the news conference, see Bell and Munro 1996; and Judy Swanson 1996. For other summaries of the 1995 and 1996 report cards, see Hay 1995b, 1996.

7 . A Canadian family is defined as "two or more people living together and related by blood, marriage, or common-law relationship" (Ross, Scott and Kelly 1996:3).

8 . A summary of the Picot and Myles research paper is in Picot and Myles 1996.

9 . A number of other publications provide perspectives on the dimensions of child and family poverty in Canada. For recent examples see: Ecumenical Coalition for Economic Justice 1996; Novick and Shillington 1996; Ross et al. 1993, 1996; Ross, Shillington and Lochhead 1994; and Scott 1996b.

10 . "A family is defined as 'poor' if family equivalent gross income is less than 50% of median equivalent gross income for the country. . . . This is a relative definition of poverty which is currently the consensus among poverty researchers conducting international comparative studies. . . . The before-tax definition of poverty . . . yields, for Canada, a poverty measure fairly similar to the Statistics Canada LICOs [Low Income Cut-offs]" (Phipps 1993:3, fn.1).

11 . Shelter (i.e., housing) costs are covered separately. An "employable" family of four in BC receives a maximum allowance of $650 for shelter (Province of British Columbia 1996c).

12 . Workers in the labour force include the employed and the unemployed. Potential workers are people who are ready, willing and able to work but are not included in labour force statistics. This is usually because these people are ineligible for employment insurance benefits or they have already exhausted benefits they were eligible to collect.

13 . Child poverty data for 1995 are not available at the time of writing.

14 . It should also be noted that family income, whatever its source, is not always shared equally within a family unit. A number of studies have examined the issues of income distribution and control within families (Cheal 1991; Eichler 1988b; Phipps and Burton 1994a, 1994b). For example, Cheal (1991) examined equality in economic "agency," i.e., independent, direct access to financial resources for three family types: breadwinner/homemaker, dual earner and dual career. Each family type was categorized by their financial resource access into either equal, low

inequality or high inequality. A slim majority (52 percent) of dual career families are egalitarian while breadwinner/homemaker and dual earner families are inequalitarian (56 percent and 67 percent, respectively). Thus, the possibility exists of a family with an adequate income containing one or more poor persons within the family (Eichler 1988a; Phipps and Burton 1994a, 1994b).

15 . As this is being written, federal and provincial ministers are engaged in ongoing talks to create a national framework for social policy, what is being described as the "social union" discussions (Greenspon 1996c). Legislated conditions for the CHST transfer *may be* one result of these discussions.

16 . For a table listing annual benefit amounts for different levels of family net income and different numbers of children, see Province of British Columbia 1996a:10.

17 . Phipps (1995b:187, fn.2) notes that, while well-being has many dimensions, her article is focused on economic well-being or material standard of living.

18 . A collection of essays by Macpherson (1987) is also illuminating on this point.

19 . I refer to voluntary organizations; business, labour and professional groups; public interest groups, churches and so on.

20 . This may not be easy, however. For example, Allen feels that "[t]he most objectionable aspect of Phipps' article is the strong assertion that children are social goods" (1995:277). Low (1996:190) neatly summarizes the underpinnings of an economic approach to social concerns as "[t]he principle of a cold calculus of individual self-interest and a belief in market forces." For a different perspective from self-described "social" economists, see Allen and Rosenbluth 1992.

21 . The five dimensions of well-being that are outlined, with associated "goals" and "requirements," are sustenance, attachments, physical and social health, stimulation and community care (Novick and Shillington 1996:7-9).

22 . For example, Kesselman concludes that cash transfers, in and of themselves, will not alleviate child poverty and that policies have to be targeted to the consequences of poverty, based loosely on the determinants of healthy child and family development (1994:87-88). This would mean that policies would very specifically target benefits and/or programs to people "at risk," or to people in particular stages of their lives. Wooley, Vermaeten and Madill (1996:24) evaluated the current federal child tax benefit and found that "few of the benefits . . . went to the poorest families . .□. because of the interaction of the tax benefit system, the greatest net beneficiaries were lower-middle income families in the $40,000 to $50,000 income range."

23 . See also Social Planning and Research Council of BC (1992) for similar arguments regarding universal income transfer programs for children and families.

Identifying Low Wage Workers and Policy Options

Clarence Lochhead

Identifying Low Wage Workers and Policy Options

In the federal government's discussion paper *Improving Social Security in Canada*, the chapter "Jobs in the New Economy" begins by stating that "the best form of social security comes from having a job" (Human Resources Development Canada 1994a:29). For the most part, this is true: unemployment is, without question, a major contributing factor to economic insecurity and family and child poverty. But unemployment and the availability of work are only part of the problem. In Canada, a substantial number of the poor (as defined by Statistics Canada's Low Income Cut-offs–LICOs) already have jobs — often full-time jobs. They are the working poor,[1] and their poverty is not the result of exclusion from the labour market, but the result of low wage work.

There are several trends which suggest that low paying jobs will become a more prevalent feature of the "new economy" in Canada: rapid growth in the number of part-time jobs and non-standard work arrangements; expansion of the low wage service sector; increasing international competition with low wage economies; continuing high levels of unemployment; declining wages among young people; and the displacement of a large semi-skilled middle class of income earners. Many of these trends and their manifestations have resulted in greater *polarization of the labour market.* As Banting, Beach and Betcherman note, "the proportion of middle income jobs, which represented the core of employment for people in Western nations during the post-war years, has declined; employment growth is increasingly found in high skill, high wage jobs at one end of the occupational hierarchy, and low skill low wage jobs at the other" (1995:1).

The polarization of the labour market suggests that low wage jobs, as a structural feature of the Canadian labour market, will have a serious and negative impact on a growing number of Canadian households. In addition to their low wages, these jobs are also less likely to provide private pension coverage, medical insurance, dental coverage and maternity benefits, to name a few. These are precisely the benefits that are increasingly important in the face of continuing efforts of governments to cut social spending. Described in this way, low wage jobs seem to have few redeeming qualities. One argument suggests that a proliferation of low wage jobs will do nothing more than create a growing underclass of working poor, substituting the poverty of the welfare cheque for the poverty of the wage, and will undermine genuine efforts to solve the problem of poverty.

A countervailing argument views low wage jobs in a more positive light. They are seen as the vehicles which provide opportunities to gain on-the-job training and work experience, and therefore serve as "ports of entry" into higher paying jobs. In other words, low wage jobs provide access to wage "ladders." And while low wage jobs may result in poverty in the short term, they provide the most promising escape route from poverty in the longer term. This is often an argument used in support of low wage job creation programs, including the recent efforts of some governments to introduce "workfare" programs.

The aim of this chapter is to identify low wage workers in working poor families, and to begin to examine their degree of wage mobility over time. Are low wage workers "trapped" in low paying, "dead-end" jobs, and thereby confined to the ranks of the working poor? Or do they experience upward wage mobility sufficient to raise them out of poverty?

The first part of the chapter identifies low wage workers using a relative (deciles) approach, and examines the demographic characteristics of those holding the lowest paying jobs in the Canadian labour market, distinguishing between low wage job holders in poor and non-poor households. The second part of the chapter considers the longer term prospects of the working poor. Using longitudinal data from Statistics Canada's Labour Market Activity Survey (LMAS), some preliminary research findings on the wage mobility of low wage workers over a three year period are examined.[2] Following the identification of low wage workers and an examination of their wage mobility, some general policy directions are identified along with a discussion of the next steps in the research.

Identifying Low Wage Workers

Low wage workers are often equated with individuals who work at a job paying the minimum wage. But this definition is far too restrictive. Minimum wage rates vary from province to province and in no way reflect the cost of living or adequacy of income. As Clark (1995) has shown, in all jurisdictions, minimum wage jobs produce incomes which fall several thousand dollars below the LICOs. A single mother and child living in a large urban centre such as Toronto or Vancouver, for example, and working at the national average minimum wage would need to work more than seventy hours per week for fifty-two weeks just to reach the poverty line (Campaign 2000 1994b). Even jobs that pay significantly more than the minimum wage can be inadequate to meet the needs of some families. For example, a father of two children whose spouse performs unpaid labour in the home could work full-time full-year at a $10 per hour job, and still have annual earnings several thousand dollars below the $25,000 poverty line. In short, to restrict the definition of low wages to the minimum wage is to fail to consider the thousands of families whose higher-than-minimum-wage jobs still result in poverty level incomes.

An alternative method of identifying low wage workers, and the one used in this chapter, is a relative approach which defines low wages in relation to the overall wage distribution. In this method, jobs are ranked according to their hourly wage rate from lowest to highest, and divided into ten equal steps or deciles. The lowest decile refers to the 10 percent of jobs that have the lowest hourly wage rates, and the top decile refers to the 10 percent of jobs with the highest hourly wage rates. These job deciles can be thought of as a wage-rate hierarchy. Low wage workers are those individuals who hold jobs at various steps in the bottom end of the wage hierarchy (for example, in the bottom 20, or bottom 40 percent of the wage distribution). While this may be a more arbitrary method of identifying low wage workers, it is a more flexible approach that facilitates greater inclusivity and comprehensiveness in the examination of (relatively) low wage job holders.

Using data from the first year of the LMAS survey,[3] the first row of data in Table 1 presents the upper limits of hourly wage rates that divided into deciles all jobs held in 1988. Upper limits are simply the highest wage rate an individual could have without moving into the next highest decile. For example, in 1988,

Table 1
Job Deciles, Hourly Wage Rates and Selected Characteristics of Job Holders, 1988

	Wage Deciles										
	1	2	3	4	5	6	7	8	9	10	all jobs
wage rate upper limit (1988$)	5.39	6.95	8.50	9.94	11.30	12.96	14.95	17.26	20.91		-
% female	61	60	58	54	54	41	34	33	27	24	47
% age 16-19	39	17	6	4	2	1	1	-	-	-	10
% age 20-24	23	27	23	19	12	10	7	6	2	1	14
% age 25-54	33	50	63	68	76	79	82	83	88	85	67
% age 55-69	5	6	8	9	10	10	11	11	10	14	9
% who are children at home	52	34	21	19	13	9	8	6	3	2	20
% head/spouse	45	63	76	78	86	89	91	92	96	97	78
% in families with earnings under $10K	25	18	13	8	5	4	4	2	2	2	10
10-20K	15	21	24	19	11	8	6	3	3	2	12
20-30K	14	14	15	20	26	27	18	9	5	3	15
30-40K	15	16	16	17	17	17	23	31	20	3	17
40K and over	31	32	32	36	41	45	50	56	71	90	46

Source: Statistics Canada, Labour Market Activity Survey, longitudinal file, 1988–1990.

the bottom 10 percent of all jobs paid $5.39 per hour or less, and the bottom 40 percent of all jobs paid an hourly rate of $9.94 or less. The top 10 percent of jobs paid more than $20.92 per hour. The remainder of Table 1 presents some selected characteristics of the people who occupy different levels within the wage rate hierarchy.

The Bottom 10 Percent: Minimum Wage Workers

All of the people in the bottom decile (jobs paying $5.39 per hour or less) were working at or near the minimum wage, which in 1988 was about $5.00 per hour in all provinces. Who are these minimum wage workers?

The data in Table 1 show that women are over-represented in the lowest paying jobs, holding 47 percent of jobs overall, but 61 percent of the jobs in the bottom decile. In addition, a large share of jobs in the bottom decile are held by teenagers (39 percent) and youth aged 20 to 24 (23 percent) which together account for 6 in 10 minimum wage workers. Over one-half of the (near) minimum wage job holders (52 percent) were young people living at home with parents. Table 1 also shows that many of those in the bottom decile live in families with relatively high earnings: 3 in 10 lived in families with annual earnings (from all earners) totalling $40,000 or more, and nearly 1 in 2 (46 percent) in lived in families with total earnings of $30,000 or more. In short, a large share of these bottom decile or minimum wage workers might be characterized as "secondary earners," that is, teenagers and young adults living at home in families with relatively high earnings.[4]

On the other hand, an almost equal share (45 percent) of those at the bottom of the wage rate hierarchy are either the head or spouse of their household, one-third are in their "prime" earnings age of 25–54, and 40 percent were in families with total earnings of less than $20,000. Overall, those with jobs in the bottom decile—with minimum wage jobs—are a diverse population, composed of individuals in both poor and non-poor families. Clearly, minimum wage workers are not synonomous with the working poor.[5]

An Expanded Definition of Low Wage Work: The Bottom 40 Percent

If the definition of low wage work is expanded to those with jobs in the bottom 40 percent of the wage rate hierarchy (jobs paying $9.94 per hour or less), the demographic profile of job holders changes in some important ways. First, there is a dramatic decline in the proportion who are teenagers. While 39 percent of jobs holders in the bottom decile are teenagers, this falls to 17 percent of those in the second decile, 6 percent in the third decile, and only 4 percent in the fourth decile. Conversely, the proportion of low wage job holders who are twenty-five years of age or older rises sharply. In addition, the proportion of job holders who are children and young adults living at home falls, with individuals who are either the head or the spouse of the household making up the majority of low wage job holders. In other words, the expanded definition of low wage work is more likely to include individuals who are the "primary earners" in their households, and who are responsible for the maintenance of the household and the well-being of the household members. Finally, the expanded definition of low wage work captures a significant number of workers whose higher-than-minimum wage jobs still leaves them with relatively low earnings. For example, 27 percent of job holders in the fourth decile (jobs paying between $8.51 per hour and $9.94 per hour) live in households with total annual earnings of $20,000 or less.

As in the case of minimum wage workers, however, not all low wage workers by this expanded definition live in "poor" families. In order to examine the problem of low wage work as it affects the working poor, it is therefore necessary to examine low wage job holders in the context of their household income.

Identifying the Low Wage Working Poor

To examine low wage workers living in poor households, both the individual's wage rate and the level of household income must be considered simultaneously. Unfortunately, the LMAS provides neither a measure of total family income nor an indicator of poverty. Despite these limitations, the survey data does include a measure of total household earnings. For the purposes of this chapter, a household with total annual earnings under $20,000 is deemed "poor."[6]

The intersection of an individual's wage rate and the total household earnings (from all members) is presented in Figure 1. Two categories of individual wage rates and three categories of household earnings are used to produce the matrix. Individuals whose jobs were in the bottom four deciles of the wage hierarchy are labelled as "low wage workers," and those with jobs in the top six deciles are labelled "high wage workers." Total annual household earnings are divided into three categories: low earnings (under $20,000); modest earnings ($20,000-$29,999); and "high" earnings ($30,000 or more). The resulting matrix yields

Figure 1: The Intersection of Individual Wage Rates and Total Household Earnings, 1988

	Total Annual Household Earnings (1988$)		
Individual's Wage Rate	Under $20,000	$20,000-$29,999	$30,000 or More
"low wage workers" $9.94/hr or less (bottom 4 deciles)	"low wage workers in low earnings households"	"low wage workers in modest earnings households"	"low wage workers in high earnings households"
"high wage workers" more than $9.94 (top 6 deciles)	"high wage workers in low earnings households"	"high wage workers in modest earnings households"	"high wage workers in high earnings households"

six possible combinations of relative wage positions and total household earnings.

For this analysis, the focus is on low wage workers in low earnings households. These are individuals whose lowest paying job in 1988 was less than $9.95 per hour (the bottom four deciles) and whose total annual household earnings were less than $20,000. This group is loosely defined as the "low wage poor." In 1988, there were 2.2 million individuals who fit this description, accounting for 17 percent of all paid workers, and 36 percent of those who held a paid job in the bottom four deciles of the wage distribution. Roughly three-quarters of the low wage poor were the head or spouse in their household.

Wage Mobility among the Low Wage Poor

While low wage jobs are inadequate to meet their immediate needs, what are the longer term prospects of the working poor? Are the low wage poor likely to remain within the ranks of the working poor over time? Or do they escape their poverty through upward wage mobility? The answer to these questions will cast new light on the extent to which job creation at the bottom end of the wage scale will contribute to the continuing persistence of poverty, or whether low wage jobs will present opportunities for real increases in standards of living.

This section presents some initial research findings on the relative wage mobility of the low wage poor over the period 1988-1990. Wage mobility is measured as an upward/downward change in an individual's *relative* position within the wage distribution. In other words, only those individuals who move from one wage decile to another are said to have experienced wage mobility. The results of this analysis are presented in Table 2, which shows the percentage distribution of low wage workers in 1988 by their relative wage position in 1990. In other words, of those workers with low paying jobs in 1988, what proportion moved up or down the wage rate hierarchy by 1990? The boldface percentages in Table 2 indicate wage stability (workers who stayed in the same relative position on the wage hierarchy), the percentages to the right of the boldface represent upward mobility and those to the left indicate downward mobility.

The first conclusion to be drawn from Table 2 is that the low wage poor appear to have experienced a considerable amount of relative wage mobility over the three year period. Of those whose lowest paying job in 1988 was in the bottom wage decile (the first row in Table 2), about one-third (34 percent) were still in the bottom wage decile in 1990, almost one-half (48 percent) had moved upward in the wage hierarchy, and 17 percent had moved out of a paid employee relation (either to self-employment, unemployment or not in the labour force).

For those in the first decile, there is obviously no measurable downward wage mobility since they are already on the lowest rung of the wage ladder. Downward relative wage mobility is observable, however, in deciles two through four, with between 12 and 24 percent of individuals experiencing a downward move in their relative wage position. Among those who experienced upward wage

Table 2
Relative Wage Mobility Among the Low Wage Poor, 1988-1990

Wage Decile, 1988	Wage Decile, 1990							No Longer Wage Labour			Total
	1	2	3	4	5	6	7 to 10	self-emp.	unem-ployed	not in labour force	
1st	**34**	18	9	7	5	2	7	3	3	11	100%
2nd	12	**26**	14	10	6	4	10	3	4	10	100%
3rd	3	12	**33**	13	7	4	7	4	2	13	100%
4th	2	5	16	**29**	14	6	12	4	2	9	100%

Notes: The wage decile in 1988 refers to lowest paying job held in that year, and in 1990 it refers to the highest paying job in that year. Low wage poor is defined as an individual whose lowest paying job in 1988 was among the 40% of lowest paying jobs, and whose total household annual earnings was under $20,000.

Source: Statistics Canada, Labour Market Activity Survey, longitudinal file, 1988-1990.

mobility, most increased their relative position by one or two steps. Overall, the prospects for upward wage mobility among the low wage poor appears to be a "mixed" story. For every ten low wage poor, about four moved up, three remained in the same relative step, one went down, and two were no longer holding paid jobs.

While it is difficult to assess whether this degree of relative wage mobility is high or low, it appears to be consistent with other studies of wage mobility among low wage workers. In a U.S. study of earnings mobility among minimum wage workers, Smith and Vavrichek (1992:82) found that over 60 percent of workers earning the minimum wage in the 1980s were earning higher wages one year later. Using a relative approach, a recent Danish study showed that less than 20 percent of individuals remained in the bottom four deciles of the wage distribution over a four year period (Westergard-Nielsen 1994). Finally, Metcalf (1981) noted considerable wage mobility among the lowest decile of workers in Britain, but cautioned against over-emphasizing this mobility since there was considerable movement in and out of low paying jobs over a five year period. The results for Canada (presented in Table 2) show considerable individual wage mobility as measured at two points in time — 1988 and 1990 — with about 40 percent of low wage workers experiencing a wage rate increase sufficient to move them upward in the wage rate hierarchy. In this sense, it is apparent that a considerable proportion of low wage workers are not "trapped" at the same wage level over time. However, it is also clear that the majority of low wage workers remained at the same level, moved down or dropped out of the labour force. In short, low wage work may be a stepping stone to better paid employment for some, but appears to hold limited opportunities for the majority. Further research is required to examine movement in and out of low paying jobs, and the characteristics of those who make positive gains versus those who do not. Some of these characteristics are presented below.

The proportion of low wage workers in poor households who experienced upward wage mobility between 1988 and 1990 appears to vary considerably in relation to age, sex and family status. Figure 2 demonstrates that young people experience greater upward wage mobility than do older workers. About one-half of teenagers and youth working in low paid jobs in 1988 experienced upward wage mobility by 1990 (Figure 2). The experience is not the same for all young workers though—men aged 20-24 are somewhat more likely than their female counterparts to have experienced relative wage mobility. The prospects for upward wage mobility are somewhat reduced for individuals between the ages of 25 and 54, with 41 percent of men and 36 percent of women having made relative wage gains. The proportion of low wage workers aged 55 to 69 who experienced upward mobility is in part an outcome of the large share who dropped out of the labour force between 1988 and 1990. Still, upward mobility among older workers, particularly among men, appears very limited.

Figure 2: Percent of Low Wage Poor* Experiencing Upward Wage Mobility, 1988–1990

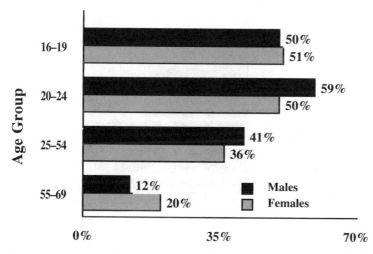

*Low wage poor are persons with jobs in the bottom four wage deciles whose total household earnings are below $20,000.

Source: Statistics Canada, Labour Market Activity Survey, longitudinal files, 1988–90.

Figure 3: Percent of Low Wage Poor Experiencing Upward Wage Mobility 1988–90, by Family Status

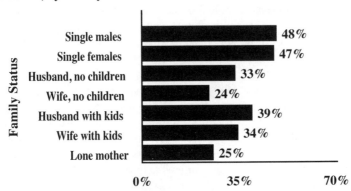

*Low wage poor are persons with jobs in the bottom four wage deciles whose total households earnigs are below $20,000.

Source: Statistics Canada, Labour Market Activity Survey, longitudinal file, 1988–90.

Figure 4: Percent of Low Wage Poor* Experiencing Upward Wage Mobility 1988–90, by Education in 1988

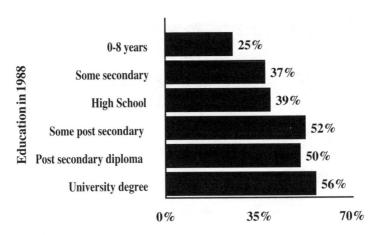

*Low wage poor are persons with jobs in the bottom four wage deciles whose total households earnigs are below $20,000.

Source: Statistics Canada, Labour Market Activity Survey, longitudinal file, 1988–90.

Figure 3 shows that the likelihood of upward wage mobility is similar for single males and single females. Women in families, however, were less likely than men in families to move up the relative wage ladder. Further research needs to explore the relationship between womens' roles in the families and their opportunities for wage mobility.

The low proportion (25 percent) of lone mothers with upward wage mobility is due in large part to the fact that 42 percent of wage-earning lone mothers in 1988 were no longer in paid labour in 1990 (either unemployed, stopped looking for work or self-employed).

Higher levels of education clearly increase the likelihood of upward wage mobility among the low wage poor. Among low wage workers in 1988 with post secondary education, over one-half moved up the relative wage ladder (Figure 4). Although not shown in this figure, this positive relationship between education and upward mobility holds true even after factors such as age, sex and family type are taken into consideration.

This rather cursory examination of factors associated with the likelihood of upward wage mobility is meant to demonstrate a simple point: to the extent that we can identify the conditions under which people are more likely to experience upward wage mobility, we can begin to understand the resources and supports required by individuals that enhance upward wage mobility. The findings in this chapter indicate that opportunities for advancement among the working poor are not an automatic or inherent feature of the jobs they hold. Without this recognition, and in the absence of policies and programs aimed at creating opportunities for advancement, any growth in the number of low wage jobs will likely contribute to a growing and permanent class of working poor Canadians.

Summary and Policy Directions

The aim of this chapter has been to identify who low wage workers are and to examine their degree of wage mobility over time. The research findings show that low wage workers are a diverse group: some support families; others are teenagers living at home; some are young adults living on their own; some are poor; and others appear to being doing well because of additional earners in the family. Because of this diversity, it is clear that low wage work does not produce the same degree of economic insecurity to all low wage job holders. Policy responses to the economic insecurity caused by low wage work should recognize this diversity with appropriately designed income security programs.

The preliminary research findings on wage mobility over the period 1988 to 1990 show a considerable degree of movement in the relative wage rates of low wage workers. It seems apparent that some low wage workers—about four in ten—are only temporarily in low wage positions, and that these jobs are simply stepping stones to higher paying jobs. On the other hand, about one-third of those with low wage jobs experienced no upward mobility, and one in ten actually went down in the earnings distribution. Finally, one in ten low wage workers had dropped out of the labour force and the remainder had become unemployed or self-employed.

The next steps in this research will be to examine the following in greater depth: the differing profiles of low wage workers and their implications for policy; the factors contributing to wage mobility; and the range and mix of policy instruments appropriate to address both issues of income security and wage mobility.

At this stage we can, at the very least, identify the range of policy instruments available and some of the considerations around each. In addressing the issue of income security among low wage workers, two primary instruments have been relied upon by governments — the minimum wage and earnings supplementation schemes. The first, the establishment of a minimum wage, seeks to provide a basic wage floor for all workers (with some exceptions). As a means of addressing the inadequacy of earnings among the working poor, the minimum wage serves a useful role but, on its own, it has been criticized as being a less than effective anti-poverty measure (Economic Council of Canada 1990; West and McKee 1980; International Labour Organization 1995).

One major criticism is that a large proportion of those directly affected by the minimum wage are not poor (Economic Council of Canada 1990). The findings presented in this paper on the income characteristics of those in the bottom decile of the earnings distribution confirm that a large proportion of minimum wage increases would go to individuals in non-poor households. At the same time, many individuals in working poor families would be unaffected by modest minimum wage increases since their wage rates can be several dollars per hour higher than the minimum standard. Increasing the minimum wage might be an appropriate response to other policy issues, but as a targeted anti-poverty strategy, it is a blunt instrument at best.

A second common criticism of the minimum wage is in relation to its supposed disemployment effects. In short, this (contentious) argument suggests that, as the minimum wage increases, it becomes more costly for employers to hire workers, therefore taking jobs away from those who are most commonly found in minimum wage jobs — the unskilled with little education or marketable experience. To the extent that this argument is true — and there are numerous empirical studies both to support and refute it[7] — minimum wage increases could close opportunities for some low wage workers, denying them access to potential wage ladders. With these and other criticisms of the minimum wage as an anti-poverty tool, much focus is now on various direct income and earnings supplementation schemes.[8]

It is not possible here to engage in an indepth discussion of the various income and earning supplementation schemes, but some general comments are worth making. Earnings supplementation schemes could make low wage work "pay" for many families whose incomes, despite their labour market participation, still fall below the poverty line. Such programs would be of particular benefit to families with children. An earnings supplementation scheme, in combination with other supports like childcare and dental coverage would go a long way to improve the financial situation of working poor families. If done in concert with a reasonable minimum wage policy (i.e. a minimum wage which reflects the cost of living of an individual worker), an earnings supplement for families would help redress the inability of the labour market to recognize the cost of raising children.

In addition to the minimum wage and supplementation programs, further policy research should work to identify the conditions and factors associated with upward wage mobility, and the supports and resources required to help low wage workers get better paying jobs. Policies that promote real opportunites for wage advancement should be an integral part of the variety of initiatives required to address the needs of the poor.

Notes

1. There is no consensus on the definition of the working poor. In the *Canadian Fact Book on Poverty* (Ross, Shillington and Lochhead 1994), the working poor are defined as non-elderly households whose adult members collectively have at least forty-nine weeks of either full- or part-time employment in a given year, and whose total income is below Statistics Canada's Low Income cut-offs. Using this definition, in 1992 there were 512,000 working poor households in Canada, making up twenty-nine percent of all non-elderly poor households. On average, these working poor households had sixty-one weeks of employment, and roughly seven in ten working poor households had at least one adult working on a full-time, full-year basis. For alternative definitions of the working poor, see National Council of Welfare (1995a); Gunderson, Muszynski and Keck (1990); and Klein and Rones (1989).

2. This research is part of an ongoing project on low wage work and wage mobility being undertaken at the Canadian Council on Social Development and funded by Human Resources Development Canada.

3. The data source for this analysis is Statistics Canada's Labour Market Activity Survey 1988-1990 (longitudinal file). This survey collected information on the wage rates and labour market experiences of 55,434 persons over a three year period.

4. Low wage jobs held by teenagers or youth in families should not be discounted as without significant consequence. For example, many of today's young people must work long hours at low paying jobs as a means of financing their post secondary education.

5. Throughout this chapter, the term poverty reflects a family-based measure of income adequacy. That is, an individual is only "poor" if they live in a poor household. Family-based measures of poverty assume sharing of resources between family members.

6. The choice of this "poverty line" is not completely arbitrary. In 1988, the Low Income Cut-off (LICO) for a family of three living in a large urban centre was $22,169. In addition, median family income in 1988 was $41,200. The $20,000 earnings cut-off used in this analysis to identify poor households is therefore

145

roughly equivalent with both the LICO and 50 percent of median family income. No effort has been made, however, to adjust this low earnings cut-off for family size. The main purpose of this study is not to provide estimates of the number of low wage poor, but to examine characteristics of the low wage poor and their prospects for upward wage mobility.

7. West and McKee (1980:99) for example state that "there is no convincing evidence to refute the prediction that minimum wages cause reductions of employment," while the International Labour Organization suggests that negative employment effects of minimum wages are "minimal" (1995:150).

8. See, for example, the Human Resources Development Canada (HRDC 1994b) background paper on guaranteed annual income.

Fighting Child Poverty with Parental Work Income Supplements

STEVE KERSTETTER

Several forms of income assistance have been proposed in recent years as part of the broader campaign to reduce child poverty in Canada. There have been proposals to restructure the federal child tax benefit to provide higher benefits at the lower end of the income scale. Ontario developed the idea of an "integrated" child benefit aimed primarily at helping low wage families with children. Still another possibility is earnings supplements for low wage parents. Earnings supplements have received less attention in social policy circles than the other two approaches. The purpose of this chapter is to describe in some detail one possible model for a work income supplement and the impact it might have. The chapter is an extension of the research undertaken by the National Council of Welfare (1994a) for a report entitled *A Blueprint for Social Security Reform*.

Work income supplements are hardly a new idea in North America, and both Quebec and the United States introduced income supplements of their own within the last few years. Quebec's Parental Wage Assistance Program (commonly known as APPORT, the acronym for the French name of the program, *Aide aux parents pour leurs revenus de travail*) included a work income supplement of up to $4,232 in 1994 for a couple with two children. APPORT also provides assistance for childcare and housing costs under certain conditions. The U.S. federal government has an Earned Income Credit with a maximum benefit for the 1994 tax year of $2,528 U.S. for a family with two children. The National Council of Welfare's proposals for a parental work income supplement borrow features from both programs.

The council sees a number of advantages in the creation of an entirely new kind of social support rather than trying to rework existing supports. The work income supplement suggested here is entirely new as it would provide income to low wage parents on top of any income they receive from existing government programs. With a properly designed supplement, all recipients would wind up with additional disposable income. No one would end up with less. In contrast, some of the federal child tax benefit options would see middle income families with children losing benefits to cover the cost of increasing benefits to low income families.

A work income supplement would help correct the inability of the wage system to provide for the cost of raising children. A nurse or a sales clerk or the proverbial rocket scientist all get paid according to salary scales which take no account of the number of dependents they support. Even with higher wages and more fringe benefits, there will always be jobs that do not pay parents enough to raise their children.

A work income supplement would help offset the disincentives to work that exist in provincial and territorial welfare programs, especially the problem of high welfare "taxbacks." Many welfare recipients lose a dollar of their monthly welfare cheques for every dollar of earnings beyond a minimal amount. No other approach to helping low income families with children has been able to address successfully the problem of high welfare taxbacks.

Nonetheless, there are two limitations to parental work income supplements and many of the other proposals for fighting child poverty that have to be acknowledged at the outset. First of all, a work income supplement has to be reasonably large to be effective, and that means it would likely be reasonably expensive. Cost is not an insurmountable problem, but it puts the onus on proponents of work income supplements or alternative approaches to show that the additional money required can be found at a time of severe restraint on government spending.

Second, while a work income supplement can provide much needed additional income to low wage parents, it would not likely lead to dramatic or even significant reductions in rates of family poverty by itself. Many poor families live thousands of dollars below the poverty line, and even an additional benefit of $3,000 or $4,000 a year is not enough to move many poor families out of poverty. This is an obvious problem for people who want to see immediate and tangible results from any major new initiative.

A Model of a Parental Work Income Supplement

What follows is a refinement of a proposal first published in *A Blueprint for Social Security Reform* (NCW 1994a). Figure A shows benefits for low wage families with one child in the top half and benefits for families with two or more children in the bottom half. The benefit for a family with one child would be 35 percent of gross earnings to a maximum of $3,000 a year, and the benefit for a family with two or more children would be 35 percent of gross earnings to a maximum of $4,000. Benefits would be non-taxable, and they would not be considered as outside income for the purposes of welfare entitlements. In other words, the supplement would not trigger cuts in a family's monthly welfare cheque. Families would receive the supplement every month, the same as the federal government's child tax benefit. To avoid unnecessary duplication, the new work income supplement would replace the supplement of up to $500 a year that is part of the existing child tax benefit.

The principal design features of the work income supplement model are a large maximum benefit, a fast phase-in rate, a long "plateau" for maximum benefits and a fast rate for phasing out benefits. A large maximum benefit is appropriate because of the huge depth of poverty among families with children.

Figure A: Model Work Income Supplement, Family with One Child

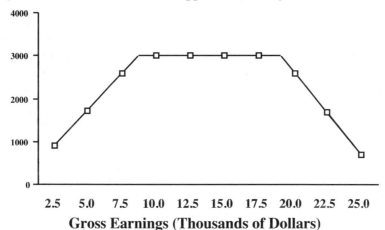

Gross Earnings (Thousands of Dollars)

Model Work Income Supplement, Family with Two or More Children

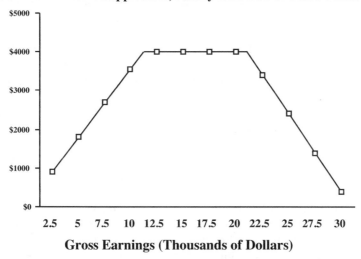

Gross Earnings (Thousands of Dollars)

The National Council of Welfare publication *Poverty Profile 1993* (NCW 1995a) reported that poor couples under 65 with children under 18 had, on average, annual incomes $7,677 below the poverty line. Families led by single-parent mothers under 65 were even worse off, living an average of $8,566 below the poverty line.

The work income supplement would be phased in quickly at a rate of 35 percent of gross earnings to ensure that sizable benefits go to parents with earnings from part-time as well as full-time jobs and also to address the problem of high welfare taxbacks for parents who have both welfare income and wage income. The plateau in the model extends over an earnings range of roughly $10,000. This would increase the number of beneficiaries overall and the number of families getting the maximum benefit. The plateau would also minimize the prospect of families having their supplements adjusted month after month because of modest changes in earnings. The work income supplement would be phased out quickly, at a rate of 40 percent of net family income, in an effort to keep the cost of the program within reasonable bounds and to target benefits to low wage parents. Benefits would disappear at net parental income of $26,500 for a family with one child and $31,000 for a family with two or more children.

The cost of the model in Figure A was estimated by Human Resources Development Canada (HRDC) as a courtesy to the National Council of Welfare. The price tag came in at $1.66 billion a year. Two other variations with the same basic design had price tags of $1.57 billion and $2.24 billion. To put these costs into perspective, an additional $1.66 billion would amount to one percent of the $164.2 billion in the federal government's main spending estimates for the 1995-96 fiscal year. If the cost was shared by Ottawa and provincial and territorial governments, the burden on any single government would obviously be much lighter. In the view of the National Council of Welfare, the best way for governments to find the extra money needed for a work income supplement or other social policy initiatives would be to eliminate wasteful tax expenditures or "loopholes" in the system. *A Blueprint for Social Security Reform* (NCW 1994) identified billions of dollars of tax expenditures which could be trimmed or eliminated outright without increasing the tax burden on low income Canadians and without subjecting high income Canadians to taxes out of line with taxes in the United States.

Another possibility is to create an entirely new tax on transfers of wealth similar to the taxes on wealth transfers that already exist in the United States. That would make Canada's tax system more equitable and could bring in extra revenues in the order of $1.9 billion a year.

In terms of the impact on families, the computer simulation used by Human Resources Development Canada estimates that the model work income supplement would benefit 934,000 low wage families with children. An estimated 369,000 families with one child each would receive $1,435 in benefits on average, with actual benefits ranging up to the maximum of $3,000 a family. The remaining 565,000 families with two or more children would receive $2,008 on average, with actual benefits ranging as high as $4,000.

The National Council of Welfare acts as a policy adviser to the Minister of Human Resources Development on matters affecting low income people. The council has never claimed special expertise in program administration or delivery. For that reason, it chose not to make detailed recommendations to the federal government on the way a work income supplement should be run. In general terms, however, the council's preference is for a supplement that would be cost shared by the federal, provincial and territorial governments and delivered by the provinces and territories through a "single window" approach. Parents who receive some welfare to augment their earned income could have their supplement payments calculated each month by welfare officials at the same time that they calculate any changes in welfare entitlements because of earnings during the previous month. Low wage parents who receive no welfare could receive their supplement cheques by mail based on their earnings during the previous year.

A program shared by the two levels of government could be fine tuned to take into account interrelationships between a work income supplement and provincial and territorial welfare programs and tax regimes. Quebec has done extensive work to harmonize the Parental Wage Assistance Program with its tax and welfare systems, and other jurisdictions would do well to follow Quebec's example.[1]

One of the chief advantages of a parental work income supplement is its ability to offset longstanding disincentives built into the welfare system, especially high welfare taxbacks. The following two figures show how this would occur. Figure B shows a "typical" welfare benefit of $1,000 a month for a single-parent mother with one child. We assumed that the welfare system has an earnings exemption of $100 a month in net earnings—an exemption that is comparable to those in use in about one-half of the provinces and territories. The single parent in the example can earn up to $100 without any reduction in her welfare cheque. However, she loses a dollar of welfare for every dollar in net earnings above $100 a month.

Figure B: Typical Disincentives to Work in the Current Welfare System, Single-Parent Mother with One Child

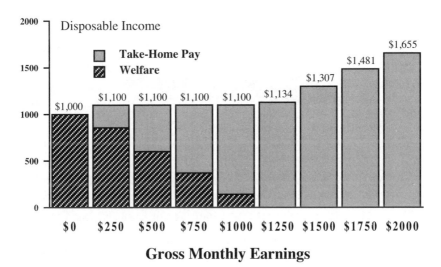

Gross Monthly Earnings

The bars in Figure B show disposable or after-tax income as the parent's gross earnings rise from zero to $2,000 a month. Each of the bars is shaded to show the portion of disposable income that comes from welfare and the portion from take-home pay—gross earnings minus income taxes, Canada or Quebec Pension Plan contributions and unemployment insurance premiums. To put the figures into perspective, gross earnings of $1,000 a month are roughly equivalent to earnings from a full-time minimum wage job.[2] The bar at the extreme left of the graph represents a family with $1,000 a month in welfare income and no earnings. The next four bars show the disincentives associated with the earnings exemption. As earnings rise and welfare entitlements fall, disposable income remains fixed at $1,100. The parent in the example can stay home and receive $1,000 a month or join the paid labour force and work 170 hours a month at the minimum wage and wind up with $100 more—a net gain of 59 cents for every hour on the job.

Some provinces have earnings exemptions that are a combination of fixed amounts plus a percentage—for example, an exemption of $100 a month of net earnings plus 25 percent of net earnings in excess of $100. This kind of exemption is fairer than a fixed exemption alone, but it still leaves tremendous disincentives to work in the welfare system.

Figure C shows the impact of the model work income supplement with a maximum benefit of $3,000 a year or $250 a month. The graph is the same as the previous one, except for the supplement shown in black. The parent working full-time at the minimum wage winds up with $350 a month more than the parent on welfare alone.[3] Because of its ability to offset high welfare taxbacks, a

Figure C: Disposable Income from Welfare, Earnings and Work Income Supplement, Single-Parent Mother with One Child

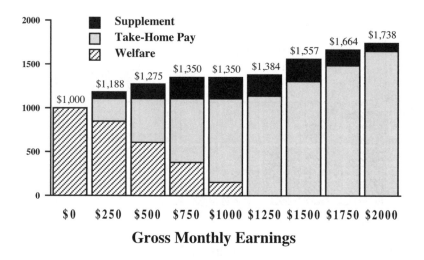

Figure D: Disposable Income from Welfare, Earnings and Integrated Child Benefit, Single-Parent Mother with One Child

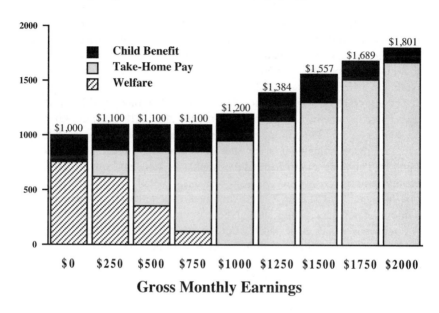

Gross Monthly Earnings

Disposable Income from Welfare and Earnings in Current System, Single-Parent Mother with One Child

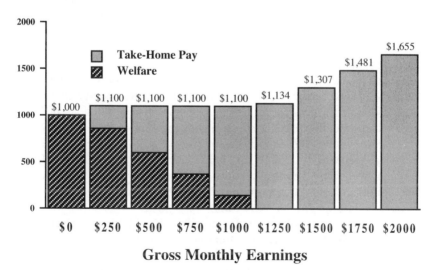

Gross Monthly Earnings

153

parental work income supplement has a clear advantage over other approaches to income assistance for families with children, including Ontario's proposals for an integrated child benefit. Ontario proposed, in effect, to remove children from the welfare rolls by converting the portion of the family welfare cheque intended for children into a benefit that would be integrated with other benefits paid by governments on behalf of children. The integrated benefit would be paid to all low income families with children—whether or not the parents received welfare.

The top graph of Figure D shows the impact of an integrated benefit on the disposable income of a single parent with one child. The maximum benefit is $3,000 a year or $250 a month—the same amount as the model work income supplement and somewhat larger than the alternatives studied by Ontario. The integrated child benefit of $250 in the graph was deducted from the amount the family had previously received from welfare, so the maximum welfare benefit is $750 rather than $1,000. The maximum child benefit of $250 was reduced at a rate of 25 percent for families with net parental income in excess of $19,000.[4]

For purposes of comparison, the bottom graph of Figure D shows the current welfare system as shown earlier in Figure B. Families who relied on welfare for some or all of their income would be no better off than previously with an integrated child benefit, and they would still face the same disincentives that they faced previously. This is evident by comparing the bars in the top and bottom graphs of Figure D. For families with gross monthly earnings up to $1,000, disposable income is the same in both graphs. The only difference is the components that make up disposable income in each case.

Disincentives in the welfare system are outlined in the report *Incentives and Disincentives to Work* (NCW 1993). The report contains detailed calculations of the take-home pay of typical households where some parents worked full-time at the minimum wage and others relied largely on welfare. The comparisons for the three types of families with children described in the report are reproduced in Table 1 for each province and Yukon. Figures were not available at the time for the Northwest Territories. All the calculations were based on 1992 data. The situation has not changed appreciably since then in most jurisdictions, but there have been major cuts in welfare rates in Ontario, Manitoba and Alberta.

The figures in brackets represent disincentives to work—where families on welfare are better off financially than families headed by parents with full-time minimum wage jobs. The figures without brackets show incentives to work—where families with parents working at the minimum wage are better off financially than families on welfare.

For the single parents represented in the table, all jurisdictions except Quebec had disincentives to work, ranging from $46 a year in Manitoba to $4,685 in Ontario. Quebec had incentives to work because of the Parental Wage Assistance Program. The report calculated that the single parent in Quebec in the table received a work income supplement of $2,870.

Table 1: Annual Incentives (and Disincentives) by Family Type, Welfare versus Work at the Minimum Wage, 1992

	Single Parent, One Child	One-Earner Couple, Two Children	Two-Earner Couple, Two Children
Newfoundland	(2,135)	(2,696)	5,022
Prince Edward Island	(2,697)	(8,080)	(312)
Nova Scotia	(2,853)	(3,717)	4,269
New Brunswick	(789)	(3,003)	4,977
Quebec	2,793	(574)	7,154
Ontario	(4,685)	(8,810)	735
Manitoba	(46)	(9,047)	(1,353)
Saskatchewan	(618)	(4,390)	2,467
Alberta	(1,815)	(7,407)	1,049
British Columbia	(2,556)	(5,572)	2,925
Yukon	(1,115)	(7,723)	1,766
(Figures in brackets are disincentives)			

With a federal or federal–provincial work income supplement of $3,000 added to the figures in Table 1, single parents with one child in all jurisdictions except Ontario would find work more financially rewarding than welfare. For the one-earner couples with children in Table 1, a work income supplement of $4,000 would turn disincentives to work into incentives in four provinces and would greatly reduce the size of the disincentives in the other jurisdictions. For the two-earner couples with children, a supplement of $4,000 would remove disincentives in Prince Edward Island and Manitoba and add greatly to the incentives already found elsewhere.

In summary, a parental work income supplement could be a vital part of a comprehensive program to reduce child poverty in Canada, but it is not a panacea. A work income supplement is not a substitute for sound economic policies, especially policies for creating more and better jobs and reducing the rate of unemployment. It is not a substitute for higher minimum wages or better labour standards. It is not a substitute for welfare reform, using reform in the best sense of the word. And it is not a substitute for affordable and accessible childcare and other social services that support low income and middle income families.

Notwithstanding these caveats, a parental work income supplement has the capacity to provide thousands of dollars a year in additional income to low wage parents. It addresses the inability of the wage system to provide a "living wage" to parents in all family circumstances. And it offsets directly the main disincentives of the welfare system that have led to a loss of public support for welfare in recent years.

Notes

1 . The impact of a work income supplement in any province or territory depends in part on the type of earnings exemptions in the welfare system and whether there are special provincial or territorial tax breaks for low income earners. Ideally, the plateau for the maximum supplement should extend up to the point where a family's entitlement to welfare disappears entirely because of other sources of income.

2 . To illustrate clearly the impact of a work income supplement, the calculations in Figure B and the rest of the graphs in this article were limited to welfare and earnings. Low income families would also qualify for the federal child tax benefit, federal GST credit, and certain other supplementary provincial or territorial benefits or tax breaks. Normally, families in the income ranges shown in the graphs would qualify for maximum benefits from these programs. The comparisons illustrated in simplified form in the graphs would not change.

3 . The fact that disposable income remains fairly flat in the middle bars of Figure C shows the need for further refinements in the design of the supplement or its interaction with provincial or territorial welfare and tax regimes. The problem could be corrected, for example, by earnings exemptions based on a percentage of net earnings rather than a flat $100, by a low-income tax credit or tax reduction or by a larger maximum supplement.

4 . To maintain consistency with earlier graphs, the value of the federal child tax benefit was not included in the calculations for an integrated child benefit. The relative differences between the top and bottom graphs of Figure D would be exactly the same if the child tax benefit was added to both.

Part 4:
Advocacy and the Politics of Influence

Advocacy, Political Alliances and the Implementation of Family Policies

Maureen Baker

Introduction

The welfare state is not just a set of programs and services but rather a system of ideas about collective responsibility, justice, equity, the family and personal responsibility (Wilson 1977; Williams 1989; Ursel 1992; Lewis 1993). Family policies, which are usually implicit within general social policies, contain ideas about who constitutes a family, what obligations family members have to each other and to government, and what rights individual family members can expect the state to protect. These ideas are often a compromise among those desired by members of Parliament, those pressed by the opposition parties and those advocated by citizens' groups lobbying for legislative change.

In this chapter, three case studies emphasize the ways in which political alliances have influenced the development of family policy in North America. The 1988 attempt to remove childcare funding from the Canada Assistance Plan, the 1990s debate over maternity leave in the United States and the present campaign to eradicate child poverty in Canada (Campaign 2000) will be discussed. These examples illustrate how alliances and political pressure not only help to reform family policies, but also work to impede change. The political context of Canada and the US will be compared to that in several other countries, as this chapter is based on a comparative study[1] of policies to reduce child and family poverty in eight industrialized countries (Australia, Canada, France, Germany, the Netherlands, Sweden, United Kingdom and the United States).

Politics and Social Policy

A survey of the development of family policy[2] indicates vast differences in the comprehensiveness and generosity of benefits for families with children (Baker 1995a). Researchers and theorists disagree over the reasons for uneven development in these different jurisdictions. Most focus on a combination of economic conditions, demographic pressures and political factors (Baker 1995a; Boreham and Compston 1992; Wennemo 1994). In this, I will focus only on political factors, especially political alliances, ideology and structures.

Political Alliances and Policy Change

Countries with strong social welfare programs tend to be those in which the prime beneficiaries of the programs have united to form effective coalitions to pressure government. Because so many groups lobby for change, politicians tend to listen to those who appear to represent greater numbers, who are apt to make their lives most difficult or who are willing and able to create alliances with a powerful political party (Esping-Andersen 1985; Kangas and Palme 1992-93).

Effective political alliances must be developed among like-minded groups and these groups need to attract the attention of politicians with power. Although groups with opposing views may try to influence politicians, the successful lobby must gather support from many different constituencies or be well funded and well organized in order to influence the government in power. Furthermore, the demands for policy or legislative change need to be perceived to be within the mandate and capability of the government to resolve.

When groups are able to create coalitions, they are more likely to gain strength and influence politicians. However, the ideology of the party in power is also important in determining to whom governments listen and which policy alternatives and outcomes they finally choose.

The Importance of Political Ideology

Many theorists argue that despite economic globalization, growing bureaucratic complexity and rising unemployment, political ideology remains the decisive factor in explaining the development of social and economic programs (Banting 1987; Boreham and Compston 1992; Väisänen 1992). Over the years, political parties were created precisely because different philosophical assumptions exist about issues such as: the role of government in personal life; how best to keep a nation and its citizens prosperous; and whether and how income and wealth should be redistributed from the rich to the poor, or from individuals or couples to families caring for dependent children.

Traditionally, Canadian political parties have supported different kinds of policies. Some parties have favoured more generous benefits to families with children, such as a universal family allowance, a refundable child tax credit and higher tax deductions for childcare. Other parties have been more supportive of policies benefitting individuals, corporations or foreign investors, including greater tax concessions for political contributions than charitable donations, a higher annual contribution level for RRSPs, and "tax holidays" for new enterprises. In Canada, the New Democratic and Liberal Parties have been historically more involved than the Conservative Party in the development of social welfare programs. In the 1990s, however, there has been considerable ideological convergence among political parties regarding a number of economic and labour issues on which they were traditionally divided. Provincial New Democratic Parties (especially in Ontario and Saskatchewan) have become more concerned with reducing the deficit, downsizing government and lowering labour costs, even though these issues traditionally were associated with Conservative ideology. The policies of the Liberal and Conservative Parties have also converged in recent years. For example, although the Conservatives abolished the universal family allowance before they were voted out of office in 1993, the federal Liberals have made no attempt to reinstate it despite earlier commitments to the principle of universality. Furthermore, the Liberals continue to cut federal transfer payments to the provinces, which fund the very social programs they created in earlier years. The most dramatic illustration of this involves the legislation of the Canada Health and Social Transfer (CHST) that replaced the Canada Assistance Plan (CAP) in 1996.

Structural Barriers to Reform
In Canada, the federal system and the division of powers between federal and provincial governments have served as barriers to the development of several social programs (Banting 1987; McGilly 1990). The introduction of unemployment insurance, for example, required an amendment to the Constitution in the 1940s because initiating an employment-related program was outside federal jurisdiction. Because so many family-related policies fall under provincial jurisdiction, the Canadian government cannot create a national program without first obtaining the agreement of the provincial governments. In contrast, countries with central governments such as Sweden and France have been able to expedite social reform favouring families and children more effectively than decentralized governments such as Canada and the United States (Wennemo 1994; Baker 1995a).

Since the early 1980s, antagonisms over constitutional reform and national unity have made policy agreements among provincial and federal governments very complex. In the spring of 1994, for example, the federal government began a contentious review of unemployment insurance and welfare programs but this was diverted by some provincial opposition, the 1995 federal budget cuts and the subsequent move to impose block funding for provincial health, welfare and educational programs. Reforming the conditions of cost shared programs (such as CAP) require federal–provincial agreement, but block funding means that decisions about the nature of social programs are left to the provincial governments with fewer federal restrictions and fewer federal dollars.

The participants of the decision making process and the legal requirements of consultation also influence which policies are deemed acceptable. In Canada, there is no formal procedure for governments to negotiate with interest groups except non-binding consultations in parliamentary committees.[3] In addition, there is no strong, visible and continuing alliance between labour unions and any federal political party that has won an election. In contrast, there has been a historical alliance between labour unions and the Social Democrat Party in Sweden and between the unions and the Labour Party in Britain and Australia.

Furthermore, many social policy decisions in Sweden are made by boards with representatives from labour, employers and government, and governments cannot make decisions without the representation and participation of these groups. In Sweden therefore, the structure of decision making, as well as coalitions and political alliances, influence the development of social policies.

Ideology, Advocacy and Political Alliances: Three Case Studies

The importance of ideology, advocacy and political alliances in influencing the development of family policy is illustrated in the three case studies looked at below. The first was an unsuccessful attempt to remove childcare funding from Canadian welfare legislation. The second examines the debate over maternity leave in the United States. The last case study considers the current Canadian campaign to eliminate child poverty by the year 2000.

The Proposed Canada Child Care Act, 1988

As more mothers have entered the labour force, most governments have acknowledged the need for preschool childcare services. The difficult political questions are who should provide these services and who should pay for them. Some see childcare for preschool children as "education" that should be regulated, subsidized and provided either by government or not-for-profit organizations. Others argue that family members or the private sector can provide childcare services with minimal government regulation and expenditure.

Although the regulation and licensing of childcare services fall under provincial jurisdiction in Canada, the federal government made provisions for sharing the cost of childcare services for low income families under the CAP beginning in 1966. Since 1971 the federal government has also provided income tax deductions for the childcare expenses of employed parents. To receive federal contributions under CAP, the provinces must spend the money first and then ask the federal government to match eligible expenditures specified in the plan. Whatever the provinces spend on eligible services, the federal government has been required to match in funding. In each province, childcare subsidies are available for some families in financial need, generally in government-regulated centres or family care homes.

Critics of childcare funding under CAP have argued that it treats childcare as a welfare issue rather than as public education or a requirement for working parents. Furthermore, critics have noted that poorer provinces do not have the initial funds to spend on childcare, that eligibility regulations for subsidies are too strict, that national standards are absent, but most of all, that subsidized and regulated childcare remain too costly and in short supply. One outcome is that many Canadian parents must rely on unregulated sitters to care for their preschool children (Canada, House of Commons 1987; Friendly 1994).

The political barriers to changing policy can be illustrated by the 1988 attempt to reform childcare funding. The proposed Canada Child Care Act attempted to remove childcare funding from CAP and to establish a new arrangement in which more costs would be shared but a spending ceiling would be placed on federal contributions. The Conservative government that proposed the bill was under growing pressure from the business lobby to reduce government expenditures and balance the budget. This lobby included the Canadian Manufacturers' Association, the Business Council for National Issues and the Canadian Federation of Independent Business, as well as conservative "think tanks" such as the Fraser Institute.

As the provinces and territories have jurisdiction over childcare, the federal government needed their support to change the legislation, especially if they wanted to give the new program national standards or objectives. Furthermore, some provincial governments would have gained more money under the new plan while the more urbanized provinces (Ontario and Quebec), had been rapidly expanding subsidized spaces, would soon have lost if the new funding formula had become law.

Parliament was expected to hear the concerns of various advocacy and cultural groups, including First Nations, unions, and childcare, feminist, "pro-family" and religious groups, before the legislation could be passed. Yet Parliament had no legal requirement to amend legislation in order to incorporate their concerns.

All groups which appeared before the special legislative committee opposed major segments of the bill. The governments of Ontario and Quebec argued that the legislation would eventually reduce federal money for childcare in their provinces. Quebec also opposed any attempt to create national standards or to attach "strings" to the transfer. The Child Care Advocacy Association of Canada opposed spending public money on for-profit daycare and argued in favour of national standards for care. The pro-family movement (including REAL Women of Canada) wanted tax credits for parents who care for their children at home. Feminist groups (such as the National Action Committee on the Status of Women and the Canadian Advisory Council on the Status of Women) and trade unions (such as the Canadian Union of Public Employees and the Canadian Federation of Labour) wanted more subsidized childcare spaces, public funding only for not-for-profit care, and better wages for daycare workers.

None of these lobby groups were powerful enough to convince the federal (Conservative) government to amend the legislation. One reason was that the impetus for this bill had largely come from the daycare lobby, feminist groups and unions, but many Conservative members of Parliament were more influenced by the pro-family movement, the business lobby and the concerns of the two largest provinces. Business groups argued that investing more government money into childcare would raise taxes, and asking employers to invest in childcare would increase operating costs and reduce profits. Second, the bill was introduced just before an election call, indicating that the government may not have intended to pass it all but rather wanted to appear reform-minded.

While the Conservatives held the majority in the House of Commons early in 1988, the Liberals retained most seats in the Senate. At that time, the Senate was being portrayed by the Conservatives and by many citizens as an appointed, unrepresentative, costly and unnecessary structure of government. The Conservatives used the childcare bill in the power struggle with the Liberal-dominated Senate and argued that the non-elected Liberal senators were preventing the Conservatives from creating a national childcare program. While the Senate was preparing to ask for reforms for the childcare bill, an election was called which automatically removed the bill from further consideration. The Conservative government then blamed the Senate for "killing" the childcare bill. Yet, after the Conservatives won the 1988 election, no new childcare legislation was introduced. Nor has any new legislation been introduced by the Liberals since they won the 1993 election.

Creating a new cost shared program requires federal–provincial consent, which appears to be extraordinarily difficult to gain at this period in Canadian history. Instead, the Liberals have announced the new CHST which will replace cost sharing with block funding to the provinces for medicare, post secondary education and social services (including childcare). Under the new CHST, the possibility of creating a national childcare program seems very remote. Provinces will acquire more discretion to create their own social welfare programs, but discrepancies among provincial childcare systems will become more apparent in the future as federal transfer payments will be reduced.

The Recent Debate over Maternity Leave in the US

While federal–provincial disputes and cutbacks impede the development of a national childcare program in Canada, right-wing ideologies and alliances have prevented the United States government from introducing maternity or parental benefits. Unlike Canada and the other countries in this study, the United States has no national law requiring employers to provide paid maternity, paternity or parental benefits. In 1993, the *Family and Medical Leave Act* required employers to provide employees with twelve weeks of unpaid leave in the event of medical emergency, childbirth, adoption or the need for dependent care. This legislation represented fifteen years of controversy, as it had been passed on two previous occasions by both Houses of Congress but had been vetoed twice by President Bush (Kammerman and Kahn, forthcoming). Yet the leave remains unpaid, and only covers employers with fifty or more employees, as well as employees with at least one year of service with the same employer.

The decision to provide maternity benefits in the US remains in the hands of employers and unions, and some provide short periods of paid leave as part of sickness or disability benefits (Lubeck and Garrett 1991). Nevertheless, there has been a lengthy debate over these policies and several earlier attempts to legislate maternity leave and benefits.

In 1978, the federal Pregnancy Discrimination Act (PDA) defined pregnancy ás a "temporary disability" that should be covered by existing sickness and medical plans (Kammerman 1991). Women working in firms that offered disability insurance had their coverage extended to include pregnancy and maternity, yet the Act did not obligate employers to provide such insurance even though most women worked in firms without it. The most important effect of the 1978 Act was to require the five states which did provide temporary disability insurance (TDI) to cover working women. Since 1978, no other states have mandated such insurance (Kammerman 1991).

In 1990, only 17 percent of employees working in small firms in the US were allowed unpaid maternity leave and in 1991 unpaid maternity leave was available to only 37 percent of employees in private sector firms with 100 or more employees (United States Department of Labor 1993:81). Paid maternity provisions are rarely found and paternity leave is not officially endorsed (Marlow 1991). Maternity and paternity leave tend to be confined only to those states with higher levels of unionization such as New York, where collective bargaining agreements entitle either parent to infant care leave for seven months on a mandatory basis and two years on a discretionary basis (Hayes, Palmer and Zaslow 1990). Yet at the state level, there is a growing movement to establish parental leave (Lubeck and Garrett 1991:197).

In US debates over parental leave, a major objection has been the assumed high cost. In 1988, the General Accounting Office estimated that it would cost US businesses about $340 million for an eighteen-week unpaid parental leave policy. The cost of extending the program to medical leave and leave for adoptive mothers and sick children was estimated at $160 million annually (Kammerman 1991). On the other hand, the US Chamber of Commerce calculated a much higher figure, estimating the cost to business as $2.6 billion to $16.2 billion a year. After publicizing these projected costs, the Chamber of Commerce was able to organize a massive campaign against legislated leave, basing its arguments on the high cost to business and opposition to government regulation (Bravo 1991).

Compared to the seven other countries (Baker 1995a), the US debate over statutory maternity or parental leave is unique in several ways. First, most of the controversy has been over *unpaid* rather than *paid* leave, despite the fact that the other countries have offered paid leave for years. France, for example, introduced paid maternity benefits in 1913, Germany in 1927 and Sweden in 1937 (Baker 1995a). Second, most of the US proposals have suggested a system administered through private insurance companies rather than the public sector, even though the other countries provide public insurance. And third, the legislation which finally passed in 1993 covers only a minority of companies while most employees work in smaller firms unprotected by the legislation (Garrett, Wenk and Lubeck 1990). Clearly, the legislation is a "modest" reform

(Kammerman and Kahn, forthcoming).

The importance of ideology and political alliances is apparent in this controversy. During the debate, US feminists (including the Women's Legal Defence Fund and the Institute for Women's Policy Research) argued that unpaid leave would benefit mainly middle class (white) and married women who can afford to be absent temporarily from work without wages (Bookman 1991). If lone-parent or low-income women were forced to accept unpaid leave, their families would fall below the poverty line and they would be forced to turn to welfare (Aid to Families with Dependent Children), which would be more costly to the government in the long term. Furthermore, feminists, unions (such as the Coalition of Labor Union Women and the Service Employees International Union) and other equal rights activists (such as the National Association of Working Women) argued that unpaid leave would perpetuate the gendered division of childcare (Bravo 1991; Spalter-Roth and Hartmann 1991; C. York 1991). Paid leave, on the other hand, would encourage equal opportunity for women by increasing their attachment to the labour force and their job seniority. Greater equality of opportunity for women could lead to promotions, higher wages and less reliance on welfare. Advocates of extended paid leave noted that it would increase the number of mothers of newborns staying at home, thereby reducing the demand for public infant care (Hayes et al. 1990).

In the lengthy debate over maternity and parental benefits, the US Chamber of Commerce led an alliance with business groups such as the American Society of Personnel Administrators and with Republican politicians against the introduction of federal statutory benefits, which were supported by the unions, social reformers and feminists mentioned above. The business lobby appealed to American values of individualism and non-intervention into employment practices by government. It argued that "government mandates deny employers flexibility and take away freedom," and "other countries that provide leave are stagnating [and] don't have buoyant job creation like the United States" (Bravo 1991:168). The business lobby also argued that if such leave were legislated, taxes would have to be raised when they were already too high. Despite these perceptions, the US had the lowest rate of income tax of the eight countries compared (Baker 1995a).

The business alliance argued that if employers were forced to pay for parental leave, the added payroll costs would negatively impact on economic productivity and global competitiveness (Bravo 1991). These arguments made an impact on Republican politicians, who ensured that the proposed legislation was "watered down" to unpaid leave required only for medium and large employers. Despite the fact that this legislation passed through Congress, it was initially vetoed by the US president.[4] It was not until the US government changed from Republican to Democrat and President Clinton came into office that the legislation was eventually enacted in 1993 (Kammerman and Kahn, forthcoming).

Child Poverty in Canada

In contrast to the right-wing coalition that successfully fought parental benefits in the US, a strong left-wing coalition is forming in Canada to pressure the federal government to reduce child poverty. In November 1989, Canada's House of Commons unanimously passed a resolution affirming that members of Parliament would seek to eliminate child poverty by the year 2000. This resolution arose from the work of several Canadian parliamentary committees, from United Nations' decisions about children's rights and from an international study revealing comparative child poverty rates (see Baker 1995a).

Since 1980, several Canadian parliamentary committees have studied child poverty and federal child benefits with the intention of restructuring them. The two main committees were the Senate Standing Committee on Social Affairs, Science and Technology and the House of Commons Committee on Health and Welfare, Social Affairs, Seniors and the Status of Women which established a Sub-Committee on Poverty in 1989-90. These committees made the political decision to use the term "child poverty" rather than just "poverty" to avoid any implications of the "deserving" poor and "undeserving" poor, and to elicit concern and willingness to act from all political parties. After all, if the focus is on children, no one can blame their poverty on laziness, lack of job skills or defrauding the unemployment system. Between 1989 and 1991, both Senate and House of Commons committees produced reports on child poverty recommending numerous policy changes (Canada, Senate 1989, 1991; Canada, House of Commons 1991).

Several activities in the United Nations also placed pressure on the Canadian government to act on reducing child poverty. The UN had declared 1979 the International Year of the Child and in 1989, ten-year anniversary statements were made about accomplishments and challenges during the decade with respect to children's rights. In addition, a UN Convention on the Rights of the Child, which is a binding international legal agreement, became effective in that year, thirty years after the UN Declaration on the Rights of the Child. As one of many countries, Canada signed this convention, which promised certain protections to children's financial, emotional and physical well-being. These UN activities placed pressure on the Canadian government to promote children's rights and resolve child poverty.

Additional pressure was placed on the Canadian government when international studies using the Luxembourg Income Study (LIS) database compared income distributions and transfers in major industrialized countries (Ringen 1986; Ross and Shillington 1989). These studies revealed that the US had the highest rate of poverty for families with dependent children in the mid-1980s,[5] and Canada was not far behind. These statistics were revealed in public hearings before several parliamentary committees and published in a book (Ross and Shillington 1989) that was used widely by Canadian anti-poverty groups (such as the National Anti-Poverty Organization and the Child Poverty Action Group).

In subsequent years, the LIS studies were even better publicized and discussed in parliamentary hearings and within Canadian government policy circles (Phipps 1993). According to various LIS papers, the rate of poverty for all families with children was 17.7 percent in Canada in 1987 compared to 25.4 percent in the United States. At the same time, Germany and Sweden have managed to keep their rates of child poverty at 8.8 percent and 4.7 percent respectively. For one-parent families, the Canadian rate was much higher at 48.8 percent, while in Sweden the rate was only 8.3 percent (O'Higgins, Schmauss and Stephenson 1990; McFate 1991; Smeeding and Rainwater 1991; Phipps 1993).

While arguing that child poverty had to be eradicated, the Conservative government in 1990 placed a five year ceiling on increases to the CAP for the three "fiscally strongest" provinces (Ontario, Alberta and British Columbia). This ceiling forced those provincial governments to pay a larger share of program costs and to reduce services. At the same time, federal transfers to the provinces for post secondary education and health, both affecting families with children, were limited in an attempt to reduce the deficit.

As part of the campaign to deal with child poverty, the Conservative government introduced a four part initiative in 1992 called "Brighter Futures" (Canada, Government 1992). The first was the ratification of the UN Convention on the Rights of the Child (but this had already happened in December 1991). The second was the new child tax benefit which was implemented in January 1993 immediately following the 1992 constitutional crisis. Formed by combining the money from the two child tax credits and the family allowance (FA) this benefit has been viewed by many critics as a regressive step. It added no new money for poor or middle income families, it is not fully indexed to the rising cost of living, and it removed the universality of the previous FA (Battle and Torjman 1993). The third part of Brighter Futures was Canada's Action Plan for Children, which provided aid to children's projects in developing countries. The fourth was the Child Development Initiative which provided $500 million over five years for children who are at risk because of poverty, ill-health, unhealthy living conditions, neglect or abuse. Yet if one calculated how much money would go to each child "at risk," it would amount to only $100 per year (Hubka 1992). When Brighter Futures was announced, no campaign was launched to fight unemployment, raise minimum wages or improve income security programs.

Despite public statements in the United Nations and Canada's Parliament, the previous Conservative government placed other priorities before the elimination of child poverty. Admittedly, it is difficult for the federal government to unilaterally reduce child poverty because many issues which cause it (such as low minimum wages, low social assistance rates and the enforcement of child support) are outside federal jurisdiction (Baker 1995a). Furthermore, poverty is largely caused by unemployment or underemployment (National Council of Welfare 1994b), and reducing unemployment is difficult for Canada when so many firms are foreign-owned and markets are outside the country (Baker 1995a). Furthermore, employment, training and education are a provincial jurisdiction.

Although researchers have argued that child and family poverty could be reduced through more effective transfer payments (Battle and Muszynski 1995; Baker 1995a), this would require strong political leadership and cost money. Finding the funds would require major changes in spending priorities, cuts to programs or revamping the income tax system. The Liberal government shied away from systematic reforms to social programs after initiating a major social security review and extensive public consultations on how it should be done. Instead, the federal government began to cut expenditures to social programs through reduced levels of block funding to the provinces and through the elimination of some tax concessions.

In contrast to the inaction of government, a growing number of advocacy groups have organized to fight child and family poverty. Since 1971, the National Anti-Poverty Organization has worked hard to eliminate poverty through public awareness, community organizing and advocacy. The Child Poverty Action Group (CPAG), established in 1985 to try to end poverty in families with children, has received financial, staff and organizational support from numerous other charitable foundations. In its first five years, CPAG issued a series of reports outlining the dimensions and impact of child poverty and proposing strategies for change (Wharf 1993b). In 1989, CPAG was instrumental in founding Campaign 2000, a national movement to build awareness and support for the 1989 House of Commons resolution to end child poverty by the year 2000 (Campaign 2000 1994c). In addition, the National Forum on Family Security, established in 1991 with financial support from the Laidlaw Foundation, argued that economic and social insecurity now permeates middle class families as well as poor families and that policy must be shifted from remedial measures to prevention (National Forum on Family Security 1993). These organizations and others have kept child poverty on the social policy agenda by documenting the impact of poverty on the lives of children and articulating the case for improved programs (Wharf 1993b).

Despite the efforts of Campaign 2000 and other groups, neither the Conservative nor the Liberal federal governments have made serious attempts to reduce child poverty or to develop universal daycare. This lack of reform is partly ideological. Some Conservatives and Reform Party MPs do not support much government "intervention" in family life unless there is a crisis or shortage of income and, when they do, it is often to bolster the patriarchal family (such as supporting the married credit or paying an income tax credit to mothers caring for their own children). In addition, most provincial governments have done little to reduce child poverty since the 1980s. One exception is the Ontario NDP government which made major reforms to the welfare system in the 1990s and attempted to reform its daycare system in 1994.

The lack of action on child poverty largely relates to the fact that creating these programs would be costly at a time of belt tightening and deficit reduction. Furthermore, resolving these family policy issues would require contentious interprovincial jurisdictional negotiations at a time of continuing national unity problems.

While many national, provincial and local organizations are concerned with the welfare of children, they tend to function in isolation from one another and from the provincial ministries that set policy and administer services. These organizations tend to lack access to the corridors of power and possess limited resources from which to advocate (Wharf 1993b). Consequently, their voices are overshadowed by the well funded business lobby arguing for deficit reduction and program spending cuts. Yet Campaign 2000 is a reflection of a growing and unified social movement to reduce child poverty.

Conclusion

In recent years, Canadian and US advocacy groups pressing for reforms to family-related programs have been relatively weak and underfunded compared to organizations pressing for lower taxes, cutbacks to social programs and deficit reduction. In the US, an effective alliance has developed between the political right and the moral right that has prevented the implementation of several pieces of legislation (or reduced their effectiveness) (Baker 1995b). The moral right, backed by fundamentalist Christian groups, has supported the patriarchal family and opposed increased rights for working women, public childcare, contraception, sex education, legalized abortion, family benefits to same-sex couples and numerous other social policies affecting family life (Abbott and Wallace 1992).

Three political traditions limit opportunities to adopt more generous family policies in the US. The first is the importance historically placed on individualism, and lack of concern for the collectivity which would allow children to be seen as a shared resource. The second tradition relates to the suspicion of government, particularly in matters perceived to be "private." The third concerns the nature of the US political process, which does not lend itself to building consensus on certain principles, such as gender equality and child welfare. As in Canada, there is no legalized forum to include interest groups in decision making, and consequently they must fight with their opponents for government attention. In contrast, Sweden's comprehensive family policy has come about as a result of its tradition of collective welfare, social democracy and strong corporatist structures which promote consensus building (Haas 1991).

In the US, there is no strong precedent for national legislation because so much family-related legislation is already under state jurisdiction. In addition, the trade union movement is relatively weak and historically the labour movement in the US has never really fought for benefits assisting working women or families (Baker and Robeson 1986). As well, the US public has never voted a social democratic or left-wing government into office but has fluctuated between Republican (very conservative) and Democrat (less conservative) governments. Of the eight countries compared, social democratic and labour parties have provided the strongest voice for social reform (Baker 1995a).

In many respects, Canada and the US demonstrate similar characteristics in the development of family policies. Yet, there are also differences in the history of social programs, the structure of government, the division of powers, the linguistic and cultural backgrounds, prevalent ideologies and the economic status of the two countries. Although it is beyond the scope of this chapter to discuss these differences in detail, Canada has retained the British parliamentary system and has made greater efforts than the US to encourage the exchange of social policy ideas with Britain and Europe. In fact, Canada developed several social insurance programs (unemployment insurance and medicare) that were closely modelled after existing British programs.

Canadian governments, like all others, have historically been more responsive to some advocacy groups than to others. Employer or business groups have successfully influenced governments about minimum wages, fiscal policy and unemployment insurance, especially during economic hard times. The medical profession, especially when they linked with hospital administrators, have had a stronger influence than other health professionals (such as nurses or chiropractors) on the development of medicare. Canadian labour unions have been less influential in formulating social policy than in some European countries, except when they threatened social unrest (during the 1930s Depression) or during labour shortages (in the 1960s). Anti-poverty and welfare groups have attempted to influence family policy with limited success, but in recent years feminist groups[6] have gained a stronger voice in policy decisions.

Since the 1970s, feminist groups, childcare advocacy groups, poverty groups and the women's shelter movement have developed greater popular support and have influenced Canadian policy decisions. In addition, lesbian and gay rights groups are becoming a powerful voice in discussions concerning how "family" should be defined and who should be eligible for family benefits. Furthermore, the growing cultural heterogeneity of Canada has encouraged stronger advocacy for policies that give greater consideration to cultural differences in family life. Yet, at the same time, an effective lobby from western-based conservative groups, aligned with the fundamentalist Christian churches, continues to promote "family values," focusing on an ideal-type 1950s-style family with a strict gendered division of labour.

Although various lobby groups are pressuring the government to make opposing reforms in social policy, there exist barriers to change that are both ideological and structural. Perhaps the most significant are the federal system and division of powers between the federal government and the provinces, which have led to years of jurisdictional disputes. Obtaining consensus from ten provinces and two territories (as well as First Nations) can be time consuming

170

and contentious. Furthermore, commitments to specific social programs have become entrenched in the practices of employers, in the minds of the public and in the legal structure of the country. Because the reform of one program impacts on all others, the very idea of change creates uncertainty and caution, especially when mistrust of politicians is as high as it is among Canadians.

In some countries, family policies have been reformed to counteract declining fertility (France), to assist mothers to enter the labour force (Sweden) or to provide state recognition of the importance of "motherwork" (The Netherlands). The US stands out as a nation that has resisted any reform involving the collective responsibility for children or the development of social insurance. Right-wing coalitions have dominated the political agenda in the US, emphasizing low taxes, reduced government intervention, self-reliance and the privacy of family.

In Canada, where the idea of social insurance and national social programs has been more acceptable, coalitions advocating stronger social programs and the elimination of child poverty have maintained their strength. Yet they too must combat the strong lobby for smaller government, less generous social programs and the reinforcement of "family values." The Liberals have shifted to the political right and downplayed their traditional support for universality and collective responsibility. With no social democratic party in the Canadian Parliament, future reforms in family policies are likely to be difficult, and at best incremental.

Notes

1. This project, funded by National Welfare Grants, was published by the University of Toronto Press as a book by Maureen Baker entitled *Canadian Family Policies: Cross-National Comparisons* (1995a).
2. These policies included social assistance programs, child allowances, tax concessions for families with children, maternity/parental leave and benefits, childcare funding and services, divorce and the enforcement of support, and selected child welfare policies.
3. From 1984 to 1990, I worked as a senior researcher for Canada's Parliament and served as the research director for several parliamentary committees. In this position, I experienced firsthand the non-binding nature of submissions from the public.
4. This could not happen in Canada because our prime minister retains no veto rights over legislation.
5. LIS uses a relative measure of poverty, the percentage of families who live on less than 50 percent of the country's median income after taxes and adjusted for family size.
6. Feminist groups include the National Action Committee on the Status of Women (NAC), Canadian Advisory Committee on the Status of Women (CACSW) and Women's Legal Education and Action Fund (LEAF). However, in recent years, NAC has had its budget slashed and CACSW has been merged with Status of Women Canada, losing its "arms length" status from government.

Child Poverty Advocacy and the Politics of Influence[1]

Susan McGrath

Introduction

This chapter is a critical reflection on the efforts of a voluntary advocacy group to both create awareness of child poverty and to press for policies that will eradicate child poverty in this country. Using as a case study the Child Poverty Action Group (CPAG), a small voluntary organization in Toronto, this chapter asks why, after ten years of advocacy, the number of poor children is increasing and the programs designed to assist families and children in poverty are being dismantled.

These issues can be best understood by assuming a three part model of society: the political, the economic and the social. The social or civil society[2] is a sphere of social interaction between the economy and the state composed of the family, voluntary associations, social movements and forms of public communication (Cohen and Arato 1992:xii). The social is recognized as a critical terrain of activity, what Honneth (1991:vii) defines as a "domain in which individual and collective actors contest competing interpretations of their collective needs and normative orientations as well the distribution of scarce social resources." The political sphere consists of political parties and government structures. The economic sphere is composed of organizations of production and distribution (Cohen and Arato 1992:ix). The media of interaction of the economy is money, of the state power and of the social or civil society communication (Cohen and Arato 1992:429-30).

The basic argument of this chapter is that the economic sphere dominated the post-Second World War formation of the Canadian welfare state and, in the seventies, moved to counter the associational activity of the social sphere that was pressuring the state for expanded social welfare programs. The first section traces how two well funded business interest groups, the Fraser and CD Howe Institutes, have dominated the public discourse and successfully influenced the state to make extensive cuts in social programs, to restructure the governance of the social policy system and to withdraw government support for social interest groups.

The second section examines how the child-centred advocacy strategy initiated by the Child Poverty Action Group was coopted by the corporate neoliberal[3] agenda to support polices that treat the symptoms of child poverty not the causes. It is further argued that there is resistance within the social sphere to the imposition of the norms and values of the political and corporate elite that

172

can be mobilized. The advocacy practices of CPAG in organization formation, coalition building and public education offer some strategies for such a mobilization.

The basic premise of this chapter is that social interest groups are essential to counter the hegemony of the economic sphere in society. The creation of knowledge is an important site of resistance and struggle (Park et al. 1993:xxii). It is a struggle for the determination of truths that are not constant but transitory and variable.

Child Poverty and the Politics of Influence

The hegemonic forces that dominate Canadian society are the political and corporate elite (Kornberg and Clarke 1992; Brodie and Jensen 1988). The social policy outcome is a liberal welfare state with means tested assistance, modest universal transfers or modest social insurance plans. Entitlement rules are strict and often associated with stigma (Esping-Andersen 1990:27). It is a welfare state that reinforces the social stratification of class, gender and racial inequality (Orloff 1993). A criticism of Canada's welfare programs is that they are socially patriarchal resulting in the "feminization of poverty" (Ursel 1992; Kitchen 1992).

When compared with welfare states that developed under a social democratic tradition, the child and family policies of Canada are found wanting. European countries with social democratic or corporatist political structures have lower rates of child and family poverty and countries such as Sweden, with policies of full employment, have the lowest levels of child poverty and the highest levels of gender equality (Baker 1995a). Esping-Andersen (1990) traces the success of the social democratic governments to strong working class movements and their capacity to form coalitions.

Jensen (1989) attributes the nature of capitalism in Canada, what she calls "permeable fordism," to the underdevelopment of our welfare state. The formation of the welfare state is based on brokerage politics between bourgeois parties with little ideology, not on a partisan cleavage between labour and capital which is characteristic of European countries. The working class in Canada never occupied a privileged position in the policy bodies of the state. The framework for social security in Canada, the Marsh Report (1975), has few political roots and continues to be largely ignored.

Canadian labour unions have historically focused on the bargaining table to negotiate benefits with little interest in non-workplace issues (Brodie and Jenson 1988). This results in child and family benefits being highly commodified, that is, they are determined by workplace attachment not by citizenship. Women's inequality in the labour market coupled with their unpaid work in the home means they experience a higher incidence of poverty than men (Gunderson et al. 1990). Although women's activism in unions is increasing, they continue to be a minority in the labour movement and their issues have long been ignored (Briskin and Yanz 1985).

In the sixties and seventies independent organizations formed to represent those voices previously unrepresented in public life, e.g., women, seniors, low- and non-waged workers and people with disabilities (Clement and Myles 1994:249). The inadequacy of social welfare programs was an issue for new groups such as the National Action Committee on the Status of Women (NAC)[4] and the National Anti-Poverty Organization (NAPO) as well as traditional social reform groups such as the Canadian Council on Social Development (CCSD) and the Social Planning Council of Metropolitan Toronto (SPCMT). The SPCMT has a long history of social policy advocacy (Wills 1995; Struthers 1994; Wharf 1992) and, in 1986, sponsored the formation of the Child Poverty Action Group.

The expansion of the social policy community included the increasing presence of business actors (Haddow 1990). However, the increased activity of voluntary associations within the social sphere put pressure on the government to improve social programs, a direction not supported by the business sector. Business federations such as the Canadian Chamber of Commerce (CCC), the Canadian Manufacturers' Association (CMA) and the Canadian Federation of Independent Business (CFIB) have long been active in lobbying government for public policies that reflect their interests.

In the seventies three new business interest groups were formed: the Business Council on National Issues (BCNI), the Fraser Institute and the CD Howe Institute. The resource base of these business interest groups is extensive. The combined 1995 expenditures for the Fraser and CD Howe Institutes was $4.3 million, the BCNI does not disclose its budget.[5] The BCNI, a coalition of the largest and most powerful 150 companies operating in Canada, is also described as the "shadow cabinet" (Langille 1988) because of its close ties with the government and its influence on government policy. Its primary objective is curbing the role and size of the state (Langille and Ismi 1996).

The Fraser and CD Howe Institutes are of particular interest because of their activity in the social policy field. Both successfully penetrated the social sphere, securing the status of registered non-profit research and educational institutions. It is a charitable organization designation that allows them to issue tax receipts for donations. The 1995 receipts for both organizations totalled $2.3 million.[6] This designation enables the most profitable corporations in the country to receive a tax benefit for contributing to organizations to promote their interests. It is a tax advantage that some social interest groups, such as NAC which represents women's organizations, are not allowed because it is deemed an advocacy organization. The charitable status and label of "think tank" obscure the role of these business interest groups as advocates for particular economic interests.

The clearly stated objective of the Fraser Institute is "the redirection of public attention to the role of competitive markets in providing for the well-being of Canadians" (Fraser Institute 1996). It is instrumental in encouraging public opposition to Canadian tax rates through its annual *Tax Facts* books (Horry et al. 1995). Its publication *Poverty in Canada* (Sarlo 1992) argues that the number of poor in Canada is greatly exaggerated and advocates a narrower definition of poverty. The incidence of child poverty is reduced by lowering the income threshold at which families are defined as poor. This strategy is adopted by the Standing Committee on Health and Welfare, Social Affairs, Seniors and the Status of Women in its report *Towards 2000: Eliminating Child Poverty* (Canada 1993). The report attacks the use of Statistic Canada's Low Income Cut-offs (LICOs) as poverty measures and proposes basic income levels more consistent with Sarlo's recommendations.

The CD Howe Institute is currently in the process of what it describes as "the most ambitious series of publications in its history" (Courchene 1994:xi). It is producing fifteen studies on Canadian social policy called "The Social Policy Challenge." This series covers topics such as workfare, pensions, unemployment insurance, housing and Aboriginal concerns. Its text on social welfare policy (Courchene 1994) recommends the abolishment of the Canada Assistance Plan (CAP), which the Liberals promptly did in their 1995 federal budget. It also suggests a clearly targeted child tax credit that limits payments to middle income families. The federal and provincial governments are currently negotiating an integrated child benefit which is expected to re-direct government funding to only very poor families. In contrast, CPAG has argued that all families with children should receive some form of social benefit.

The business sector also pressures governments to reduce expenditures on social programs in order to reduce the deficit and the debt. Deficit reduction is part of the dominant ideology which is essentially about "lowering our expectations of what a society can do for its citizens" (McQuaig 1995:5). The 1995 federal budget (Canada 1995) focused on reductions in social programs leaving the tax expenditures, which benefit corporations and higher income Canadians, largely untouched. The Fraser Institute gloated about the "dramatic effect" of its 1994 conference "Hitting the Wall: Is Canada Bankrupt?" on the content of the 1995 federal budget (Fraser Institute 1995) as, it argued, the cuts in the 1996 federal budget are the same as those proposed by the Institute (Barlow 1996).

The institute further argues that there should be no government transfers to non-governmental organizations (NGOs). A policy of defunding NGOs, started by the Mulroney Conservative government, is being completed by the Chrétien Liberal government. National, voluntary, social interest organizations such as NAPO and CCSD were established with the assistance of federal government funding. The purpose of funding the voluntary sector is ostensibly to increase citizen participation. However, Loney (1977) identifies it as a government strategy to re-incorporate potentially dissident groups into mainstream society.

In the 1990s, the federal government appears to be no longer concerned about the potential of disruption by social interest groups, perhaps because it is confident that business interests will dominate the discourse of the social sphere. In other cases groups which advocate policy perspectives contrary to those of the political and economic spheres are disparagingly labelled "special interest groups" and government funding support is being withdrawn. The CCSD, the National Council of Welfare (NCW), NAPO and NAC have all had significant cuts in their funding (Cardozo 1995) and others, such as the Canadian Council on Children and Youth (CCCY), have closed down. The government is continuing to refuse core funding to NGOs. The organizations can apply for funding of projects that are consistent with government program priorities. This move completely erodes the financial stability and autonomy of these organizations.

Social interest organizations are continually challenged to secure adequate resources. Although CPAG appears to have the opportunity of five year core funding from the Trillium Foundation, there is the risk that the conservative Ontario government may interfere with the allocations to this foundation from provincial lottery funds. In the prevailing free market political culture, groups are expected to raise their own resources as evidence of the commitment of the membership. This approach ignores the fact that low income groups do not have the same capacities of higher income groups and corporate organizations. For example, membership fees for NAPO are set at $2 and $5 while CD Howe Institute members pay between $2000 and $25,000.

Popular sector groups are competing with each other for voluntary donations to replace lost government revenues. Policy and planning activities have less visibility and appeal than direct service activities in the health and social service fields. A lot of organizational time can be spent identifying potential donors such as foundations and developing proposals for funding. Part of the challenge is to re-create organizational activities so that they are consistent with the potential funders interests without losing organizational integrity. Private sector funding tends to be more time-limited because funders want to be able to respond to new requests for support. They also seek projects that will enhance their public image.

Colwell (1993) documents the close association of the foundation world with wealth and power in the United States and the conservative influence that is exerted on funding decisions. Elites are not about to support projects that expose their hegemonic influence and call for the redistribution of their wealth.

These social and business interest organizations are competing to frame the public discourse on needs determination and the allocation of resources. The difficulties in arousing public interest in social issues are enormous. Edelman (1988:7) describes the public as "a black hole into which the political efforts of politicians, advocates of causes, the media, and the schools disappear with hardly a trace." Issues have to be presented in terms that entertain, distort and shock to extract a public response of any kind. Saul (1995) argues that the ideologies of individualism and corporatism that are promoted by the economic sphere lull the general populace into a state of unconsciousness.

Business interest groups enjoy a high profile in the conservative mainstream media. For example, in an examination of sources quoted for *Globe and Mail* articles during a two year period in the 1990s, Campbell (1995) identified the Fraser Institute as having the highest number of mentions (130), followed by the CD Howe Institute (39). Organizations with a collectivist orientation receive little or no coverage. The Canadian Centre for Policy Alternatives had 18 mentions and none were identified for the CCSD. CPAG was not mentioned in Campbell's article. The limited resources of social interest groups means a limited capacity to compete within the domain of the social or civil society for public support, particularly when the primary means of public communication are controlled by business. This is exacerbated by major cuts in government funding for the Canadian Broadcasting Corporation, the media institution that is publicly-owned.

The dominance of the economic sphere is reflected in changes in government policy structures and processes. The initial development of the post-Second World War Canadian welfare state was under the direction of federal and provincial bureaucrats particularly in the poverty policy field. The details of the 1966 Canada Assistance Plan were worked out by federal staff of the then Department of Health and Welfare and their provincial counterparts on a sub-committee of the then Canadian Welfare Council (now CCSD) (Haddow 1990).

In the 1970s the state policy making capacity was significantly eroded because the authority for poverty issues was dispersed among a number of conflicting federal and provincial bureaucratic interests. The bureaucratic structure was re-organized to facilitate government-wide policy coordination, and government-funded advisory groups such as the National Welfare Council (NWC) were established (Haddow 1993). Under the federal Conservatives of 1984 and 1988 the locus of responsibility for social policy was steadily shifted from Health and Welfare to the Finance Department (Moscovitch 1990). By the late 1980s, Finance's Social Policy Division had become an active policy maker in its own right, selectively using the tax system as a mechanism for meeting social policy objectives (Haddow 1990).

In the 1990s, Canadian social policy is being completely reformed by the Finance Department (Battle and Torjman 1995). The Canada Health and Social Transfer (CHST) announced in the 1995 federal budget is a watershed in the history of Canadian social policy. It represents a withdrawal of both federal dollars and federal presence from provincially-run health, welfare and post secondary education programs (Battle and Torjman 1995; Yalnizyan 1995) and jeopardizes all attempts to reduce and prevent child poverty (Freiler 1995).

Federally there is no strong opposition voice committed to collective policy strategies. The Bloc Québécois, although social democratic in its political ideology, is committed to the separation of Quebec from the federation and on principle does not support any federal policies. The Reform Party's social policies are even more anti-collective than the current Liberal government. The New Democratic Party does not have official opposition status because of its low number of seats in the legislature. There is a small group within the Liberal caucus that supports a stronger federal role in social policy but it appears to have little or no influence.

The respective roles of the federal and provincial governments in Canadian social policy are being strongly debated. A report of the Ministerial Council on Social Policy Reform and Renewal (1995) (a committee of provincial social service and intergovernmental ministers) challenges the use of federal spending power to dictate program design as the federal government does with the Canada Health Act and did with the Canada Assistance Plan. The provinces are calling for major decisions in the design, financing and delivery of social programs to be made cooperatively by federal and provincial governments. The federal government is viewed as one of the players at the table with the ten provinces and two territories. In the area of social services, the report calls for a strong federal role in the provision of necessary income supports and a strong provincial/territorial role in the provision of human services.

The communique released after the 1996 premiers' conference identifies child poverty as "one of the most critical social policy issues facing Canada today" and "the best candidate for substantial improvement through interprovincial cooperation" (Premiers' Conference 1996:2). The social services ministers have been directed to develop a proposal for an integrated child benefit that "could be implemented within existing fiscal frameworks." This suggests that there will be no new funding and the child benefit will be cobbled together from federal and provincial funds already dedicated to alleviating poverty. This is consistent with Courchene's (1994) recommendation from the CD Howe Institute.

The weakening of national standards, shared decision making and the shift of responsibilities for social policy to the provinces raises concerns for the quality, quantity, consistency and accessibility of social programs across the country. The devolution of social policy is a challenge for advocacy groups with limited resources who have traditionally focused their energies on the federal government in Ottawa. Influence would need to be exerted on thirteen different governments.

The focus on child poverty and a child benefit is an apparent achievement for CPAG and its coalition partners. The issue of child poverty is on the public agenda and one of CPAG's original policy proposals, a national child benefit, is being considered as a solution. However, the funding being recommended is far less than CPAG's proposal and there is no evidence of the rest of the policy framework necessary to seriously address child poverty. This "cherry picking" of policy proposals by social interest groups while ignoring the whole tree is consistent with the historical relationship of social interest groups and government policy makers (Haddow 1990). The current policy direction raises concerns about a child-centred advocacy strategy.

The Child Poverty Action Group and Child-Centred Advocacy Efforts

In April 1986 the Child Poverty Action Group[7] — a public interest, advocacy and research body committed to eliminating child poverty in Canada[8] and ensuring that all children in Canada have equal life chances for their development (CPAG 1986:i) — was launched. Similar advocacy organizations have evolved in the United States (Children's Defense Fund) and in Britain (Child Poverty Action Group). CPAG does not claim to speak on behalf of poor children and their families, but argues that the well-being of children is in the interest of all members of society.

The founding members of CPAG deliberately chose a child-centred advocacy strategy in an attempt to bring public awareness to the poverty being experienced by Canadian families. The identification of poor children allowed for a construction of the chronic social problem of poverty which would hopefully resonate with the public and create support for more extensive and responsive policies than traditional anti-poverty arguments. The focus on children seeks to avoid the dichotomy of the "deserving" and "undeserving" poor which has been part of social policy debates. Children cannot be seen to be responsible for their poverty. However, even this perspective has its blind spots. Child poverty is often reframed as child neglect which re-casts the blame on the failure of mothers rather than the economic and structural conditions that give rise to poverty.

Research shows that the solutions to child and family poverty lie in a combination of child-centred programs, labour market strategies, taxation policies and government priorities (Baker 1995a; Kitchen et al. 1991). CPAG consistently promoted a combination of full employment policies, income security programs and community support services with particular emphasis on income security. The group also argued that public policies should prevent not ameliorate child poverty, and advocated policies that protect modest income families so that they do not fall into poverty.

CPAG has historically called for a universal, horizontal benefit that recognizes public responsibility for the care of children and the additional costs that all families incur by raising children. Canada currently provides the lowest basic child benefits to median income families among major OECD countries (Campaign 2000 1994c). CPAG modified its original policy platform of a universal, child income credit into a progressive children's benefit that retains a universal component with a tax credit and includes a variable, non-taxable benefit directed at families below the median income level (CPAG 1994). It argues for the doubling of federal child-related expenditures from $10 billion to $20 billion (which is 3 percent of GDP) (CPAG 1994).

The shift to a modified universal policy reflects the pressure to remain relevant in the changing policy environment. Groups such as NCW, NAPO and the Caledon Institute have all accepted a universal program as too expensive and support targeting resources to the poor although their proposals call for new monies. None of the other current proposals for a national children's benefit (Canada 1994; Courchene 1994; Battle and Muszynski 1995) support universal programs and advocate selective programs that target benefits to low income families.

Battle and Muszynski (1995) writing for the Caledon Institute (a privately funded non-profit organization) acknowledge that Canada is alone among advanced industrial nations in not providing tax relief for all families with children. They argue, however, that in times of insufficient public funds the first priority for child benefits is to strengthen income supports to poor families. They suggest that the existing federal child tax benefit and provincial welfare payments on behalf of children be replaced with a single, integrated benefit payable to all low income families regardless of their source of income—wages or welfare. The integrated benefit is intended to provide incentives to low income parents to work rather than rely on welfare to provide for their children.

Battle and Muszynski's (1995) income threshold for receiving the maximum benefit is low and, given the disparities in welfare allowances among the provinces, some parents on social assistance may receive less than they do under current programs. If implemented, the cost would be covered by the federal government and is estimated to be $2 billion over current expenditures on children's programs by Ottawa and the provinces. This is the model currently under review by the federal government. Given that the government is expected to call an election next year, there may be support for this expenditure to demonstrate that the government is responsive to an issue that is of concern to most Canadians. It is a political strategy that may successfully obscure the fact that it is government economic and social policies that are contributing to the problem of child and family poverty and that, as an isolated policy, the integrated child benefit will be woefully inadequate.

In proposals drafted for the CD Howe Institute, Courchene (1994) also suggests that Ottawa should focus on income supports for children and leave the responsibility for poor adults to the provinces. While he does not give specific numbers, Courchene proposes that the existing child benefit income threshold be reduced by thousands of dollars and that a low income, anti-poverty, refundable tax credit be created. Courchene's proposals call for a re-targeting of existing resources where modest income families would lose benefits in order to provide slightly higher entitlement to the lowest income families. He is also opposed to universal childcare, suggesting instead childcare subsidies that are income tested (Courchene 1994:81).

Children's benefit proposals have been criticized for a variety of reasons. For example, anti-poverty groups are concerned that the amounts will not be adequate and the benefit will be used to justify cuts in welfare and employment insurance and will promote the cheap labour of parents (Swanson 1994). It is expected that the proposed child benefit will not improve the income of families on social assistance: the provinces will cut their current rates by the amount of the benefit, thus transferring the welfare costs of children to the federal government. By ostensibly getting the children off welfare, pressure is then put on parents to get off welfare and into the workforce even at low wage jobs.

Kesselman (1994) is critical of family income support programs, arguing that additional cash transfers on their own will do little to arrest or reduce future child poverty. He calls for more sophisticated and targeted services for poor children and their families with economic incentives used to ensure participation. Examples are programs to reduce the incidence of low birth weights or to target expectant mothers who are drug- or alcohol-addicted. However, this service response is directed at alleviating or lessening the negative impacts of child poverty rather than eliminating it.

The need for a service response is echoed by Keating and Mustard (1993:99) who suggest that, because of poor economic growth and massive government debt, "it will be difficult to prevent many children from being caught up in poor social environments with inadequate nurturing." They argue that in a period of diminished resources the focus should be to maintain a good social environment for children at risk. Preschool programs that stimulate child development are recommended. Again, this policy emphasis gives rise to programs that are more consistent with the residual policies of a liberal welfare state and are more likely to be accepted in the current policy environment.

This shift of social policy to poor children or "children at risk" is not limited to Canada but is a growing trend in all countries creating new forms of social regulation (Lesemann and Nicol 1994). Children are deemed to be a private responsibility of parents and the state claims non-interference in the private lives of individuals (Lesemann and Nicol 1994). We see a nostalgic reconstruction of the traditional family, "an ahistorical amalgam of structures, values, and behaviours that never co-existed in the same time and place" (Coontz 1992).

The state intervenes only when parents are deemed to have failed to provide for their children and the programs are aimed at "fixing" the children. Child poverty is re-framed as child neglect. Poor mothers are characterized as "bad mothers," a distorted perception which only serves to reproduce the conditions of poverty and marginalization (Swift 1995). Social problems and social unrest are blamed on the changing nature of the family rather than as a result of governments, big business, economic changes or massive historical changes. There has not only been a feminization of poverty, but a feminization of social problems more generally (McDaniel 1993).

A child-focused advocacy strategy has been coopted by the neoliberal agenda supported by the corporate sector. CPAG has responded by shifting to a family-focused advocacy strategy. In 1994, in collaboration with the Social Planning Council and the Family Service Association of Metro Toronto, studies documenting the increasing economic and social marginalization of young families were released (CPAG et al. 1994a, 1994b). CPAG is currently developing a study of "working families" (CPAG et al. 1995). It is an attempt to connect with mainstream families who are also experiencing economic and social insecurity and to mobilize their support for family-friendly social policies. Esping-Andersen's (1990) research shows that the broader the base of who benefits from social policies, the broader the base for political support to keep them.

CPAG's materials are directed at educating the general public on the issues. The hegemony of the economic sphere is being countered by mobilizing the social sphere. Valpy (1993) argues that there is a will for solidarity and community in Canada that needs to be aroused. Recent research by the Canadian Policy Research Networks (CPRN) (Peters 1995) concludes that Canadians do not want to retreat on the social policy front. We want to participate in ongoing discussions to determine the core values that should guide the social policy process and be the benchmark on which they are evaluated. Thousands of Canadians participated in the public consultation on social policy in 1994 (Pulkingham and Ternowetsky 1996a:4), the vast majority calling for retention of a social safety net. A July 1994 Angus Reid survey indicated that 89 percent of Canadians believe that child poverty is a priority which the federal government must address (CPAG 1994).

There is, however, a profound gap on values between the general public and elite decision makers in Canada (Ekos 1995). Elites were more concerned about economic issues than humanistic values and the opposite was true for the general public. The general public supports a more interventionist government than that preferred by elites. The challenge for social interest groups is to tap into these values of humanism and citizen participation.

Habermas (1996:367) describes the core of the social or civil society as "a network of associations that institutionalizes problem solving discourses on questions of general interests." These organizations are not conspicuous in the public sphere dominated by the mass media and large organizations but "form the organizational substratum of the general public of citizens . . . who seek acceptable interpretations for their social interests and experiences and who want to have an influence on institutionalized opinion- and will-formation" (Habermas 1996:367). CPAG represents such an association.

The activities of CPAG and its partners in organization formation, network building and public communication are directed at mobilizing the social sphere. In its membership and organizational structure, it is consistent with social movement organizations (Offe 1985; Adkin 1992). It has consciously chosen not to institutionalize itself through incorporation as an expression of confidence that poverty can be eliminated along with the need for the group itself. The organization consists of a steering committee of middle class professionals with some attachment to the welfare state. A core of activists have remained relatively consistent over the life of the group, providing organizational continuity and interorganizational linkages that have provided important support in terms of resources and legitimacy. Staffing is provided on a part-time basis either in the form of in-kind services or funded according to available resources. It has a close working relationship through staff and board linkages with the SPCMT and the Family Service Association.

Advocacy groups such as CPAG are basically in the business of knowledge creation which relies heavily on expertise. The ability to retain skilled volunteers and the contribution of in-kind services by larger organizations has enabled CPAG to operate with a modest budget.

Decision making is based on a consensual model. The small size of the organization means it has the potential of being more flexible and responsive than larger, more institutionalized groups. The lack of dependence on government funding has given the organization an autonomy in advocacy that many social policy groups have not enjoyed.

The informal institutional structure, a small constituency base and limited resources have meant that CPAG has had a modest role in the poverty policy community. Other social interest groups such as CCSD, NAPO, the Canadian Centre for Policy Alternatives and the Caledon Institute have more developed policy capacities and closer linkages with federal politicians and bureaucrats. NAPO also has direct linkages with poor people. These groups are located in Ottawa which facilitates access with each other and with the federal government. CPAG remains a Toronto-based organization with linkages with individuals in Ottawa and other social interest groups through Campaign 2000.

A strong social sphere requires a network of associations and a capacity for public communication (Habermas 1996). Network building has been a constant activity of CPAG. Collaboration can optimize limited resources and the networks formed become mechanisms for information gathering and the distribution of public education materials. In 1988 it initiated the formation of the Child Poverty Coalition. This included the following national organizations: the Canadian Council on Social Development, the Canadian Council on Children and Youth, the Canadian Child Welfare Association, the Canadian Institute of Child Health, Family Service Canada and the Vanier Institute of the Family. A number of these groups were members of an earlier coalition, the Social Policy Reform Group (SPRG) that was formed in 1984 in response to the policy proposals of the new Conservative government (Moscovitch 1990). The coalition produced a series of fact sheets entitled *A Choice of Futures: Canada's Commitment to Its Children* (Canadian Child Welfare Association et al. 1988).

In November 1989, to commemorate the retirement of Ed Broadbent (the leader of the New Democratic Party), the House of Commons passed an all party resolution to eliminate poverty among Canadian children by the year 2000. The commitment became the organizing focus of CPAG and the policy advocacy groups. In 1991, the Child Poverty Coalition expanded into Campaign 2000, a cross-Canada coalition of national organizations and community groups committed to promoting and securing the full implementation of the federal government's resolutions. Campaign 2000 has grown to a membership of fifty groups that represent national, provincial and community constituents (Campaign 2000 1995a).[9]

In 1994, in addition to its joint research study with SPCMT and FSA, CPAG worked with SPCMT and Citizens for Public Justice to develop *Paying for Canada* (CPAG, Citizens for Public Justice and SPCMT 1994). The document identified how the federal government could reduce its expenditures in its 1995 budget by the designated $8 billion without cutting social programs. *Paying for Canada* became the focus of an advocacy campaign that expanded to include numerous social justice and faith groups and seniors organizations. The campaign was unsuccessful but the process created valuable linkages and developed skills in grassroots organizing.

Although getting a network of associations to agree on a shared policy perspective is difficult, on July 1, 1994, *Investing in the Next Generation, Policy Perspectives on Children and Nationhood* (a bilingual public education document) was released by Campaign 2000. The choice of Canada Day for the release of the document was a deliberate strategy to promote social policy as a unifying force in an unstable economic and political environment. CPAG had the lead in writing the document, which attempts to refute some of the assumptions being promoted by the prevailing neoliberal paradigm around employment, the role of social programs and dependency.

Public education is a critical component of a mobilization strategy. In 1992 the first annual report card on the status of child poverty was released by Campaign 2000 on the anniversary date of the House of Commons resolution. The November date continues to serve as a focus for public education events on the status of child poverty and the impact of changing government policies. The report cards are compact and visually attractive with extensive use of graphs and images to make the information accessible to the broader public. Metro Campaign 2000, a coalition of Toronto agencies, has also released annual report cards on the status of children in the Toronto area.

Electronic communication skills are also being developed. Campaign 2000's 1995 report card was also released in a ten minute video format to facilitate coverage by the electronic media. Videos will often receive repeated showings by local cable companies and are popular with educators. The 1994 research report on the dimming prospects of young families has also been adapted into a video format.

Although the mainstream media may not be supportive of improved social policies, there are a number of progressive journalists across the country who are concerned about these issues and maintaining relationships with them is an essential part of an effective communications strategy. Early analyses of emerging policy issues is important in trying to influence the public discourse. In early 1996, CPAG was "leaked" a copy of the then unreleased report of the Ministerial Council on Social Policy Reform and Renewal. The organization developed a brief analysis of the implications of the devolution of social policy and circulated it with copies of the leaked report to policy colleagues and the media. The story was picked up by several newspapers and journalists and made the front page of *The Globe and Mail* and the *Toronto Star*.

Organizational maintenance, coalition building and public education require resources. Sustaining a coalition requires dedicated staff. CPAG provided the initial staffing support to Campaign 2000 but, by the end of 1994, CPAG's funding was exhausted. In January 1995 the other partners of Campaign 2000 organized to assume the support of the coalition. CPAG and Campaign 2000 continue despite limited and tenuous funding.

The withdrawal of public funding is placing more and more NGOs at risk and it is doubtful that sufficient voluntary donations can be raised to sustain the current system. As funding is cut, organizations are pressured to focus on their own priorities and forego collaborative strategies. However, the survival of social advocacy groups may lie in the formation of new organizational structures such as Campaign 2000 that involve the pooling of limited resources. A new collective project of social justice groups and the trade union movement may evolve. At the local level there is considerable collaboration; for example, a trade union activist sits on the steering committee of CPAG. However some union leaders want to use labour's new sense of grassroots urgency to create their own power bases and to exert their political influence through their traditional alliance with the New Democratic Party (Ziedenberg 1996). The potential for collaboration of various social movements is a matter of ongoing debate (Leys and Mendell 1992; Carroll 1992; Offe 1985; Cohen 1985). The effective countering of the hegemony of the economic sphere will require extensive networking and coalition building.

Organizationally CPAG appears to have achieved its objectives. It has produced research on the causes and consequences of child poverty. Specific policy proposals have been proposed as solutions. Public awareness of child poverty has increased. The group has worked with other organizations with similar aims and has lobbied politicians and their advisors at all levels of government. However, the organization's goals are even more elusive than they were in 1985. Child poverty is on the public agenda but the solutions to child poverty have not been politically supported. CPAG is shifting its policy focus to families and, together with its partners in Campaign 2000, is working to create more accessible public education materials. Whether their efforts will be successful in countering the hegemony of the business sector is unclear. What is clear is that, if the economic sphere continues to dominate Canadian public policy, the incidence of child and family poverty will increase.

Conclusion

This chapter attempts to explain why, after ten years of advocacy for social policies to address child poverty, the number of poor children in Canada is increasing. A three part model of society has been used to illustrate the dominance of business interest groups in both the political and social spheres. The child-centred advocacy strategies used by advocacy groups such as CPAG have managed to put the issue of child poverty on the public agenda, but not the necessary policies. The strategy has inadvertently supported the position of business interest groups that seek to reduce the role of government in social programs. The result has been major cutbacks to social programs and policies designed to support children and families. The neoliberal ideology promoted by the corporate sector seeks to privatize the responsibility of children with the state intervening only when children are deemed "at risk." Public social problems are blamed on individual failures. Moreover, the issue is gendered: "bad mothers" produce poor children.

Despite these setbacks, it is argued that social interest groups have an essential role to play in achieving child and family policies that will eliminate poverty. Although their presence is tenuous, they continue to struggle to create alternative knowledge forms that will resonate with the public and create political momentum for change. Social interest groups such as CPAG are essential democratic forms of public participation required to challenge the hegemony of the business/economic sector.

Notes

1. I would like to acknowledge the support and contributions of Christa Freiler of the Child Poverty Action Group throughout the writing of this paper and the thoughtful comments of Ernie Lightman and Rosemarie Popham on earlier drafts. Special thanks to Jane Pulkingham and Gordon Ternowetsky for their helpful advice and editing.
2. Civil society has a long history in Western political thought and has been revived in recent years as a possible response or solution to the dramatic changes the world is experiencing. See Cohen and Arato (1992) for a comprehensive, political theoretical analysis in support of civil society, Wood (1990) for a socialist critique, Tester (1992) and Seligman (1992) for sociological critiques. Putnam's (1993) research on Italian regional governments makes the link between dense associational relationships in a community and the strength of democratic practices and economic development. I have explored the role of civil society in the context of the Canadian welfare state (McGrath 1995). For the purposes of this chapter, I consider the terms "the social" and "civil society" interchangeable.
3. Neoliberalism justifies social expenditures as an investment in people not as a benevolent response to need. Work, efficiency and international competitiveness are hallmarks of this welfare state which marginalizes those who are unable to work: the young, the old and those who are unemployable for a variety of reasons (Blau 1989).
4. For a compelling analysis of the history of NAC, see Vickers et al. (1993).
5. The BCNI companies have assets of over $1.2 trillion, earn annual revenues of $400 billion and employ 1.3 million Canadians. The organization has a staff of fifteen and its budget is "secret" (Langille and Ismi 1996). The CD Howe Institute spent over $1.8 million in 1995 and reported an accumulated net revenue of almost

$700,000 (CD Howe Institute 1996). The 1995 expenditures of the Fraser Institute were $2.5 million with net assets of $1.7 million (Fraser Institute 1996).

6. In 1995 the CD Howe Institute provided charitable receipts of $1.2 million to the corporations for their annual membership fees which vary from $2000 to $25,000 (Callender 1996) and the Fraser Institute receipted $1.1 million, most of which came from corporate foundations (Weller 1996).

7. The British Child Poverty Action Group was the organizational model. A history of the British CPAG is provided in McCarthy 1986.

8. The group has recognized this goal as the ideal, and internally viewed a child poverty rate of 5 percent as achievable.

9. For a detailed description of the formation and advocacy strategies of Campaign 2000 see Rosemarie Popham, David I. Hay and Colin Hughes, "Campaign 2000 to End Child Poverty: Building and Sustaining a Movement," in a forthcoming publication on community development in Canada, edited by Brian Wharf and Michael Clague and published by McClelland and Stewart.

"My Kids Come First": The Contradictions of Mothers' "Involvement" in Childcare Delivery

SUSAN PRENTICE AND EVELYN FERGUSON[1]

Introduction

> The kids are my world; the kids come first. If I can do something to make them happier or better, then in any way that's what I want to be doing.[2]

Those are the words of a mother we interviewed as part of a research project designed to explore the views of mothers using licensed childcare for their preschool children. With theoretical interests in a gendered and class analysis of citizen participation and control in human services, we began this study wanting to distinguish between parental involvement and control. We predicted that mothers would distinguish between forms of involvement that gave them control (over policy and other institutional concerns) and forms of involvement that allowed them to participate in the daily experience of their children. What we found indicated that control was not a meaningful axis of maternal concern for most mothers, at least as expressed through traditional forums such as boards of directors. Instead we discovered that mothers' forms of involvement have two roots: one form emerges as an aspect of over-feminization linked to the norms of good mothering; and the other form is shaped through the different entitlements that "client" and "consumer" mothers experience. Drawing on Fraser's (1989) work, we define "consumer" mothers as those women who pay full fees and who exercise market choice in their daycare selection. In contrast, "client" mothers must prove their continuing eligibility for full direct subsidies under provincial regulations.[3]

Despite an apparent consensus on the obvious "good" of parent involvement, there is virtually no empirical or theoretical research which even addresses the views of mothers on the issue (Shimoni 1992; Doherty 1991:78; Mayfield 1990). In a recent review of the literature on parent involvement in childcare one author concluded: "The need for parent involvement in day care centres seems to be based more on the beliefs of many professionals that this is an important process rather than on empirical findings. It seems particularly important to find out how parents wish to be involved" (Shimoni 1992:91). To remedy both the empirical and theoretical gap, we set out to ask mothers what they thought.

In the spring of 1994, we interviewed forty-nine Winnipeg mothers of preschoolers using licensed childcare centres to explore how they subjectively experience their use of, and participation in, childcare services. Through open-ended interviews lasting between one and two hours, we asked mothers to discuss their views of involvement and control and we analyzed these interviews both quantitatively and qualitatively. We expect that our findings express the views of more "involved" mothers; we know, for example, that our sample over-represented highly educated mothers. For these reasons, and because the sample was small, our findings should not be taken to be representative of all mothers using preschool licensed care. Despite these limits (perhaps because of them) our study reveals some remarkable patterns and provides many provocative directions for future research.

This chapters explores three interrelated findings. We found that traditional liberal democratic theory indicating the use of a board of directors as the primary vehicle for consumer participation and control was problematic for our mothers. The majority had never voted for their board and rarely saw it as a vehicle to promote their own interests. Second, mothers' perceptions of involvement in a daycare centre, a highly emotional and at times irrational process, seem strongly tied to the institution of motherhood, a phenomenon we label "the motherhood mandate" (Rich 1977; Russo 1979). In myriad ways mothers articulated the overriding importance of the daycare centre in their lives. Finally, we discovered that subsidized ("client") and unsubsidized ("consumer") mothers have sharply differing patterns of volunteer participation. Additionally, low income mothers (those who received a daycare subsidy) report that they have greater concerns about their children than full fee paying mothers. These subsidized mothers also volunteer substantially more time at their daycare centre.

In this chapter, we explore the complex multi-faceted relationships between these findings. In a world which tells all women that their children are their first priority, we seek to explain how and why "client" and "consumer" mothers respond as they do to the subtle but persistent pressure to be involved in their childcare centre.

Parent Involvement

Shimoni's (1992) comprehensive review of the parent involvement literature argues that it has been characterized by often conflicting desires: parent education, parent influence or control over quality, and parent monitoring to ensure continuity of service. Mayfield (1990) draws on Gordon et al. (1979) to describe six different types of parent involvement in early childhood education programs. *Parents as audience* represents minimal participation and involves parents listening and observing and includes open houses, children's perform-ances and newsletters. *Parents as adult learners* describes many parent educa-tion programs on topics such as child development and child management techniques. In a similar vein *parents acting as teachers of their own child at home* represents active parental participation with their children in programs such as infant stimulation, reading programs etc. A fourth level, *parents as volunteers,* includes a range of service delivery activities, in which parents act in an unpaid capacity. *Parents as paraprofessionals or paid workers* includes similar activities as above but here parents receive remuneration. Finally *parents as decision makers* describes policy making activities such as participation as board members.

Historically, "parent involvement" has emphasized parent training. Early child study specialists insisted on the reconstitution of parenting practices as a condition of using the creche (Prentice 1993; Strong-Boag 1982; Varga 1991). Second, "parent involvement" has been a goal for professionals who seek to encourage client interest in their children. For example, one early childhood educator notes that "parents who expect only a minimum of service, such as custody and socialization, are unlikely to involve themselves deeply with agency policy making in order to raise the quality of service" (Handler 1973: 275). Such thinking underlies the requirements imposed by US federal funding agencies for daycare centres to involve parents as a condition of receipt of federal funds (Shapiro 1977). Throughout the 1960s "war on poverty," expert assumptions of inadequate parenting found expression in (mostly American) "HeadStart-style" childcare programs, which made the hollow promise that better parenting could alleviate poverty and other family distresses.

But professionals have not been the only advocates of parent involvement. For nearly twenty years, childcare activists have called for community-based services with "parent participation" as a crucial element in high quality licensed childcare (Schulz 1978; New and David 1985; Ferguson 1992; Prentice 1988). The state has also acted to institutionalize parent involvement. In Canada, several jurisdictions encourage parental involvement through legislation (Friendly 1994). Some even make "parent participation" mandatory: in Manitoba, for example, a minimum of 20 percent of the seats on the board of directors of a licensed non-profit childcare centre must be held by parents (Manitoba 1982). It is important to note that there are few other social services where the involvement of participants is mandated.

The Board of Directors: Democracy and Control in Service Delivery

The most common vehicle of parent involvement in daycare delivery is the board of directors which has philosophical roots in liberal democratic assumptions about representation and control. The "board" is a longstanding element in the social service field, historically dominated by charities, social service professionals or a combination of both. Since the 1960s, charity and professional control have come under criticism from radical social workers and social movement activists who seek to empower and democratize services (Wharf 1979; Buchbinder 1979; Wineman 1984; London-Edinburgh Weekend Return

Group 1979). Their shared concern is "consumer control": the creation of political structures within agencies to permit consumers/clients to shape services in ways that better meet their real needs, as defined from the perspective of clients themselves.

In many ways, childcare services would appear to be in an enviable position with regard to consumer control. The most common form of licensed daycare delivery in Manitoba is through a centre legally managed by a board of directors where parents must hold at least 20 percent of the seats (Friendly 1994). Provincial legislation makes this form of delivery mandatory for all non-profit centres (Manitoba 1982). In Manitoba's legislation, both the charity and the professional control model are addressed: parents *must* make up a minimum of 20 percent of the board, and staff *cannot* make up more than 20 percent. Thus, the legislation works to increase parent representatives and to limit professional monopoly. Boards of directors are the most highly-placed decision makers and authority within a centre, and mandatory parent involvement would seem to ensure parent concerns would be represented. Certainly, compared to profit-making childcare centres, which lack a board of directors and which are operated as a straightforward business, a parent minority on a board does significantly improves the chances that parent concerns will be addressed. Manitoba's requirement for parent participation is widely hailed as one of the progressive features of this province's childcare system, although we see legislated "voluntary" involvement as paradoxical.

But representative structures of all kinds are under increasing scrutiny (Findlay 1993). There is a growing consensus that representative structures are actually fundamentally *unequal:* some interests are more represented than others (Mahon 1977). Problems plague small scale groups as well as the state. Representative democracy must always be organized: who will be the "representers"; how will they be selected; what is their accountability to those they ostensibly "represent"; and will the representative structure prohibit or discourage participation from those who are not officially designated as "representatives"? These apparently philosophical questions become starkly real when we consider the relationship between the representative structure (the board) and the daily experiences of the children and parents who use the daycare centre.

Findings

Our first set of findings revealed some astonishing contradictions with respect to the parent board model. Only one-third of the mothers in our sample had ever voted in an election for board membership. Given that the authority of the representative is conferred by the act of being selected by the people whom she/he is to represent, the low percentage of our mothers voting seriously problematizes claims that daycare boards are representative and hence democratic. Either board members are elected by a small minority of parents and/or there are significant numbers of appointments and acclamations.

Our finding that mothers rarely vote challenges the selection process for board membership. But we also discovered that boards, however established, rarely function as intended. The board is designed to be a resource for parents, a site of impartiality and fairness to which parents can turn if they have concerns or complaints about the centre or its operation. Yet only 37 percent of the mothers we sampled reported that they had ever approached a board member about an issue. Crucially, almost one-half of the mothers we surveyed indicated that they would "not be willing to tell a board member if they had a concern or a problem"; instead, mothers overwhelmingly report they would take their concerns to the paid daycare director.

Parental reluctance to speak with the parent board about parent concerns is compounded by the fact that very few mothers, and only one-half of the board members, report that they know what is going on with their board. Nevertheless, it is common for these mothers to preface their answer with a disclaimer that they are very satisfied with the centre notwithstanding. One mother put it this way: "I feel my daycare's doing a good job, so I really have a hard time imagining what I'd do if they weren't and how much I'd input if things weren't going the way I want." A significant minority of the mothers reported that they did not even know there was a board. While the mother who said "I have no idea who's on the board, why it's there or what it does for that matter" is probably not typical, her experience is not infrequent. Another mother explained:

> Because it's our children in the daycare, I think we should be coming to the decisions that are going to be concerning our child's daily lives in the daycare and we should have a voice in the process. And have our voices heard. But the problem is it's only the parents on the board who have their voices heard. It's not a very democratic process.

The minority of mothers who were willing to use the board tended to be board members themselves or have close personal relations to board members. One reason for this is the slippage between the identities of "board member" and parent. "As a board member and friend of board members," explained one mother, "the discussion gets blurred." Another mother, a lawyer who was not currently a board member, illustrated identity ambiguity in a story about a strict food policy at her daughter's daycare centre:

> Indirectly, I talked to other mothers at a birthday party or something. I think it was more or less private bitching amongst ourselves. It's very difficult to remember how all this happened because Dan works with all these people, so you're out socially and you talk about the daycare and some of them might be on the board, but I know it did get changed. Lots of us were unhappy with it.

While this mother was pleased that the policy changed, the salient point here is that she did not use the board as a formal resource, even though (as a lawyer) she was ideally placed to appreciate the board's formal role. Another mother who reported that she "basically knows what happens," says it is because, in addition to reading minutes, "I'm good friends with a lot of people who are on the board, and when we go to birthday parties we discuss what was said at the board."

As might be expected, board members were more likely than non-board members to report that they knew what was going on at their board, although five mothers who had sat on boards also reported not knowing or not being sure. A few mothers described the atmosphere at their centres as "hush hush." One board member said, "I feel like I'm in the dark—the director and the chair have a close liaison, and don't tell us the whole story"; others say that, despite reading the centre's newsletter or attending meetings, they do not know what is happening. Another mother, asked if she would have ever taken a concern to a board member, said "I might have and not known it. Directors usually sit on the board, don't they?"

Those mothers who report they are informed about what is happening at their boards tend to be board members, ex-board members or friends of board members. While these informal routes probably work well for some parents, informality contradicts the stated purpose of formal representation. For example, six mothers reported that while they might have been willing to talk to board members, they did not know who board members were—a damning problem for a structure attempting to "represent" parent concerns.

If parents do not vote for their representatives and have rarely taken concerns or issues to them (nearly one-half report that they would never approach a board member and do not know what is going on with the board) it is difficult to argue that the board is a significant resource for most parents. Given these limits, it might appear to be a contradiction that 75 percent of the mothers in our survey believe that parents should hold the majority of seats on a board. They explain that parents, children and family are the ones most affected by board decisions. As one mother put it:

> It's our children that are at the daycare, and I think that we should have the major decision making. I mean I don't think we should be that involved in the day-to-day running, but on the big issues, I think parents should be the ones to be heard.

Other mothers explain that "with parents involved, it doesn't get too bureaucratic," and that since "it's parents' kids they should have a say in how things are done." One woman commented, "I wouldn't want my daughter in a place where I felt out of control or couldn't suggest or change anything that bothered me." Over 80 percent of mothers report that they personally would be willing to sit on the board of directors, even though many mothers express concerns about how little time they have. They say it would be "good to know more," that they "should" be involved and that it is "important to take an interest."

Overwhelming parental willingness to sit on the board is only one way in which mothers express an interest in greater involvement in their childcare centres. Not one of the mothers we interviewed said she wanted to do less for her centre, and a great many expressed the wish to "do more."

"I Wish I Could Do More": The Motherhood Mandate

Two-thirds of the mothers we interviewed reported that they are satisfied with their level of involvement in the daycare centre. When asked, however, what would make them more satisfied, most said that greater involvement would make them happier. Over one-half said that what would make them more satisfied would be to have "more time" for the centre. Only 20 percent said that "nothing" could make them more satisfied. Mothers frequently expressed a desire for greater involvement, even when such a comment was a counter-factual response to the open-ended question posed to them by interviewers. Echoing a common theme, one mother blurted, "If I didn't work, I'd be at the centre every day." Another offered, "If I didn't have to work, I would be at home with my kids." A painful theme which emerged unmistakably from the inter-views was that, at the same time that mothers long to "do more," they are equally clear that there is "no time."

Many mothers we interviewed talked about their "time crunch." Mothers explain that they are not as involved as they wish because they have no time. Between jobs and other demands, there is less opportunity than most mothers would prefer for their centres. Despite their time crunch, however, mothers make their volunteer work with their daycare centre a priority. Even when they are involved with other groups (such as sports or recreation, professional groups, community organizations, religious or ethnic associations, etc.), 73 percent ranked the daycare centre as "most important," with another 22 percent reporting it as "somewhat important." Only 4 percent of mothers say the daycare is the least important group in which she participates. One mother put it this way: "the daycare is essential to our well-being. Other groups would be optional, things I do for my entertainment." Similar views are common. Mothers articulated these ideas in many different ways: "my kids come before my community and before myself"; "because my kids are there. My children are my first priority"; "it's my daughter's future; it's the most important place we go"; "because my kids come first; it involves them"; "I'm not involved in other groups and more involved in my son's life and this is my priority. I have a vested interest and need to put his needs before my own"; "my child takes priority more than something I would do for myself."

Even mothers who are very active volunteers (such as board members) report that they wish they could do more for the centre. For example, the chair of one board of directors, a single mother, explained how she was always searching for ways to spend more time at the centre:

> I think I've been able so far to be as involved as my time will allow, it's flexible that way. There's always something that can be done at the centre, so when I have a bit more free time, then I can offer that time to the centre.

From the perspective of liberal democratic theory, mothers who are involved as board members are fulfilling their duties as "citizens," and should be satisfied with the knowledge that they are doing so. While the liberal model presumes that the "representative" is fulfilling her mandate by acting as a representative, few of the involved mothers demonstrated this satisfaction.

So why do so many involved mothers indicate that they want to do more? Although women's paid labour is a necessary part of most families' finances, and despite the sociological reality that there are more mothers in paid employment than not, mothers with paying jobs still experience themselves as not doing what they "should" be doing: mothering. Some of our mothers express this indirectly and others are explicit. For example, one mother notes, "If I didn't have to work I would be home with my kids."

The imperative that mothers should be a mother at all times persists, even during the hours that children are in daycare. One mother expressed her frustration when she felt this was not appreciated by her daycare:

> I almost sense this feeling of, well, you've relinquished that control by putting your child in daycare and these are the consequences you've got to suffer. 'What, you want is to put your child in daycare, *and* have a say in the daycare process?' No, you're giving up that privilege.

Thus, working mothers subjectively experience themselves as not doing what they ought to be doing: namely, caring for their children. This belief is often confirmed by others.

As feminists, we assert that daycare cannot be understood outside the all-pervasive context of motherhood. We see motherhood as both an institution and a personal experience: intensely personal and subjective, produced through historically specific political and structural forces (Rich 1977; Russo 1979). When motherhood is grasped this way, it becomes easier to see that "parent involvement"—which many mothers apparently freely offer—is compelled by requirements of normative good mothering. We hypothesize that mothers' involvement in daycare delivery mediates the contradictions of being a childcare-using mother: she might be supplementing her maternal labour with paid caregivers, but at least she is helping to make that centre a caring place for her children. Hence, a longing for "greater involvement" in their child's daycare centre is a way for mothers to fulfil their desire to work while simultaneously remaining connected to their children, thus confirming that they are responsible good mothers. As one mother put it, "Fixing the environment or you know, just helping out, just coming in one afternoon a week, just so you're more involved, you don't feel so remote or alienated."

Mothers explain that the reason they cannot be doing what they "ought" to be doing (caring for their children) is because they are working. Many mothers said they wished that they did not have to work as much as they did precisely so that they could be with their children more. Yet the imperative that they ought to be with their children full-time is also a burden. For instance one mother commented, "I work and I wonder why" and, later in the interview, "I wish I could be there every day. But I can't." For these mothers, "being too busy" to be involved with their daycare centre, yet still "wishing they could be involved," is a way to mediate the desire to be more connected to the centre. The paradox, however, is that no matter how involved a mother may be in her centre, she could always be doing more. It is only from this perspective that we can understand how it is reasonable for mothers to report that their level of participation is "not enough," even when they have weekly and sometimes daily involvement. In the end, the motherhood mandate is insatiable.

Consumers and Clients

Contemporary childcare services are framed as both a welfare service for clients and a respectable market service for consumers with the former receiving means tested subsidies and the latter paying full fees.[4] In 1992 in Canada the percentage of families using licensed daycare who received direct subsidies varied widely by province from a high of 76 percent in Quebec to a low of 9 percent in Prince Edward Island (Childcare Resource and Research Unit 1993). Nationally, 44 percent of families using licensed child daycare received a direct subsidy for the spaces for their children. In Manitoba 51 percent of families received subsidies (Childcare Resource and Research Unit 1993).

This client/consumer distinction often has unacknowledged consequences for human services like childcare (Fraser 1989). While "consumers" can do whatever they wish, since they are rights-bearing purchasers, "clients" are more problematic. The hegemonic client paradigm draws on the social work tradition of the "deserving" family, where eligibility is strictly determined. This stigmatized welfare model is stubbornly impervious to advocates' efforts on behalf of its alternative: services patterned on a belief in collective provision and social responsibility. Consumers have an entitlement to service, clients are supplicants for service (Fraser 1989). Our most provocative findings reveal that "client "and "consumer" mothers do not experience the motherhood imperative similarly nor involve themselves in their centres to the same extent. We discover two unequal forms of parent involvement and two different levels of concern about their children in the centre. Whereas rational democratic discourse might predict higher income, partnered mothers to be more involved than subsidized single mothers, we find the opposite.

According to our survey, consumer mothers (twenty-three of the interviewees) are less involved with their daycare centre than client mothers (twenty-five of the interviewees). Subsidized low income single mothers spent more volunteer time, making up the bulk of mothers who report they have weekly or twice-weekly involvement; full fee paying mothers are much more likely to report once a month contributions. Not surprisingly, mothers who receive a full subsidy are much more likely to have an income below $25,000, to be living without a partner, and to be renting or living in some kind of arrangement other than owning a home.

No other variables were found to be related to mothers' self-reported levels of involvement at their daycare centres. Educational levels were not related, probably because of the relatively high number of students in the sample. Working status as full- or part-time was not explored in this study because the vast majority of mothers report working/studying full-time and correspondingly pay for full-time spaces. Levels of work/study satisfaction were not explored but might be relevant in further research.

Subsidized low income single mothers are not only more involved in their centres, but also are more concerned about their child/ren at the centre than higher income partnered mothers. Table 1 shows that mothers receiving a direct full subsidy are much more concerned about their children at their centres than fee paying mothers. The survey also suggests that concerns are related to mother's income levels and, to some extent, partnership status, with mothers without partners showing more concern than mothers with partners.[5] Levels of concern do not seem to be related to any of the other variables looked at in this study.

Table 1
Concern about Child at the Centre versus Mother's Subsidy Status

	Concern about Child at Daycare Centre		
	Yes	No	Total
	n (%)	n (%)	n (%)
Subsidized	17 (68)	8 (32)	25 (52)
Fee paying	6 (26)	17 (74)	23 (48)
	23 (100)	25 (100)	
n=48, 1 missing case			

These findings are revealing and warrant further research. Subsidy status, income and partnership status (all indicators of class) are important factors influencing how mothers experience their childcare centre. Our survey shows that low income subsidized mothers, frequently unpartnered, participate in childcare delivery more often than high income partnered and full fee paying mothers. Mothers who are positioned as "clients" (by virtue of receiving a full subsidy) are more likely to have concerns about their children and to have high levels of involvement in the daycare centre; mothers who are "consumers," (by virtue of being fee paying), have fewer concerns about their children in the centre and are less involved.

These findings suggest that all mothers experience a complicated set of feelings about using childcare, but that they respond in two distinct ways. Our major finding is that the "client" mother, with more concerns about the centre, becomes highly involved, devoting much unpaid labour and energy, while the "consumer" mother is more detached, participating at a lower rate. In a world that tells women that their children are their first priority, mothers respond differently to the motherhood imperative.

The reasons why mothers respond differently to the motherhood imperative are difficult to pinpoint. We can speculate on multiple possibilities, based on the open-ended responses from our interviewees, the relationships demonstrated by our findings and our theoretical orientation.

The fact that "client" mothers are both more involved and more concerned about their children suggests that they participate more *because* they are more concerned. Research into quality of daycare (Doherty 1991) documents widely varying ranges of quality in centres and thus emphasizes the importance of parental monitoring. "Client" mothers may be heeding this advice more carefully than "consumer" mothers. Why these mothers are more concerned is less clear from the data. However theoretical discussions of social policy (Fraser 1989; Wineman 1984) and the history of daycare (Shapiro 1977; Prentice 1989) clearly suggest that low income single mothers and their families are at greater risk for stigmatized judgmental treatment from daycare staff than mothers and children in more conventional and affluent two parent families. "Client" mothers may feel this vulnerability and opt to be more involved both to reassure themselves and to ensure protection for their children.

A second possible explanation relates to the enjoyment mothers gain from social connections made through the daycare centre. In the open-ended responses, a number of mothers comment on their enjoyment of pot luck suppers and other social and fund-raising occasions when they meet with other parents and their children. Other research confirms the importance of social support established through childcare centres (Baker and Warnyca 1996). Possibly "client" mothers experience the daycare centre as a more valuable social support and thus are more socially invested in the daycare centre than "consumer" mothers.

Another possible explanation may relate to the satisfaction mothers gain from motherhood versus their work, as well as the internal pressure to conform to the motherhood mandate. As single mothers, "clients" may feel the motherhood imperative even more strongly than "consumer" mothers. Single mothers may feel that their children receive less parenting and, therefore, that they have more responsibility. Or possibly, "client" mothers have jobs or activities that provide less personal satisfaction for them than more affluent "consumer" mothers and consequently spend more time at the daycare, a place that complements and enhances their primary satisfaction, mothering.

A fourth possible explanation rests on the logic that "consumer" mothers feel more entitled not to be involved in the centre than "client" mothers. As the recipients of direct subsidies covering their childcare costs, "client" mothers may feel that they owe the centre some of their time and energy, a form of "shadow payment" for their subsidy. While almost none of the mothers report direct pressure to participate, in a situation where some involvement through board membership and fundraising is normative, "consumer mothers" may feel more entitled to resist this expectation or at least to be content with providing the minimum. In contrast, "client" mothers may feel that they should exceed it.

Finally, both theory (Ferguson 1991; Baines, Evans and Neysmith 1991) and our data suggest that mothers are involved in their centres to "make the centre a caring place" for their children, not primarily to wield power and influence policy through board involvement. Mothers participate to ensure there is more attention for their children during field trips, to buy more toys or better food, to donate special skills to projects, to organize social events for children and families, to help with the daily care and to give more time to their own children. Mothers report being more satisfied when they are involved. They feel they know more about what happens to their child and feel they have contributed to that experience.

Why then should "client" mothers feel this differently than "consumer" mothers? There is no easy answer to this question. We speculate that "client" mothers have fewer market options, less choice about which centre they use and would have more trouble switching centres if difficulties arose. Consequently they want to be present to prevent problems, to gain some "brownie points" should their child need their intervention and to "smooth the waters" if conflict should arise. Alternatively "client" mothers probably have a different history and experience with professional caregivers, may share fewer childrearing norms with them, and may be less comfortable with experts and professional care than more affluent mothers. Parental involvement at the centre "de-professionalizes" the atmosphere and makes it less institutional, and thus more appealing to "client" mothers.

Untangling the reasons for these findings is complicated and beyond the scope of this project. No doubt a complete explanation for differential participation of "client" and "consumer" mothers involves many of the above speculations and possibly others. Whatever the reasons, the findings themselves are provocative and important and warrant further research.

Conclusions

There are multiple roots to mothers' apparently unproblematic "involvement" in daycare delivery. In addition to the above speculations, there is also the social link between gender, status and caring work, consumer control and local democracy, professional norms of "good parenting" that coax greater parental involvement in a project to professionalize parenting and, in some jurisdictions, state-legislated mandatory participation. Without attending to these multiple roots, we misunderstand how and why mothers participate as they do. Most importantly, our study demonstrates that mothers' subjective assessment of their experience is key to explaining their participation and is tied to their experience of motherhood. Just as the women's movement has maintained that "the personal is political," we assert that mothers' feelings and practices are a clue to the social organization of childcare, which can be traced through "parent involvement " (Hoschild 1983:11).

For these reasons, we see "parent involvement" as an aspect of childcare politics. Our concern, however, is not reflected in the discourse on service delivery and parent involvement. On the contrary, childcare delivery and parent involvement is represented through a remarkably apolitical language. While the class dimension of childcare—like many social services—is obscured in this language, its truly remarkable effect is the neutering of an ineluctably sexed service (Prentice 1988). Childcare services are almost always used to replace maternal labour in the home (Ferguson 1991). Evidence that childcare services substitute for mothercare is encoded in legislation which stipulates that childcare subsidies are only available if (both) parents work or study more than twenty hours a week. While full fee paying parents are free to use childcare services for any reason, the vast majority do so because mothers have paid employment.

However we also discovered through this research that class shaped how a woman reconciled herself and her involvement in the daycare centre in relation to the motherhood imperative. Our findings show that, while all mothers "want" to be involved in their childcare centres, involvement is significantly higher for "client" than "consumer" mothers. The discourse of "parent involvement" homogenizes parents, transcending particularities of class, race, sex or other identities. Thus, one effect of the language of "parent involvement" is a confounding of the client/consumer distinction. Given the widespread social assumption that children are always their parents' responsibility, "parent involvement" is a normative imperative for all parents, clients and consumers alike. In this context, there is both an internally and externally generated pressure on most parents to maximize their involvement in daycare as in other aspects of their child's life. With respect to daycare delivery, if parents are "involved" in the administration of the service, then they would seem to be positioned as decision makers with authority. As such, they could hardly be considered to be supplicants for service. Alternately, if parents are *required* to "voluntarily" participate, then parental involvement might mean something quite different. Under these circumstances, "voluntary involvement" might be a kind of parental "shadow payment"—an unacknowledged but real time/energy expenditure by parents as part of the exchange for the care of children (Hoschild 1983).

The motherhood imperative drives all mothers to want more involvement. "Client" mothers, paradoxically, respond with greater volunteer participation than more privileged mothers. We asked mothers if they had ever been coerced into volunteerism that made them uncomfortable. Most mothers said they had not been pressured formally. Based on our analysis, however, we argue that personalistic coercion is unnecessary: the whole institution of motherhood and mothers' expectations of themselves pushes them to be involved. Each mother who volunteers or chooses not to volunteer is individually struggling for a personal resolution to a political problem. Hence each portioning of time and energy is provisional, as is the resolution of these competing pressures.

Since time is a precious resource for working mothers, might there be forms of parent involvement that work more optimally? We believe there are, and mothers we interviewed provide a creative range of alternative forms of participation. Certainly, based on our findings, we believe that the model of board membership as the vehicle for parental participation is partial at best. By neglecting the complex affective dimensions of parent involvement, formal structures like the board are blind to other axes of power and tension. The board, designed to meet parent concerns, can come to be experienced as a barrier to participation—as several of the mothers we interviewed poignantly grasped.

When we began our research with mothers, we wanted to distinguish between parental involvement and control. We predicted that mothers would distinguish between forms of involvement which gave them control (over policy and other institutional concerns) and forms of involvement which allowed them to participate in the daily experience of their children. Originally, we were puzzled by research findings that indicated that control was not a meaningful axis of concern for most mothers. Instead, mothers devote their time, energy, skills and creativity towards making their centre a "caring" place (Ferguson 1991).

Through women's unpaid emotional work at a centre, they help to mediate structural contradictions. "Client" and "consumer" mothers experience these contradictions differently and tend to develop different, although parallel, strategies to mediate these contradictions. Few mothers talk about their volunteer work in this way. But when we stood back from the individual stories, we watched a pattern emerge. The pattern is one of simultaneous resistance and accommodation to the norms of "good mothering," as mothers use their volunteer labour to create the best—although always conditional and provisional—private solutions to the contradictions of public care.

Notes

1 . We would like to thank the University of Manitoba and the Social Sciences and Humanities Research Council of Canada and SSHRC Women and Change Network grant #816-94-003 for support of this project. Earlier versions of this paper were presented in April 1995 to the seventh Annual Conference of the Manitoba Child Care Association in Winnipeg, and in June 1995 to the seventh Annual Canadian Social Welfare Conference in Vancouver BC. Thanks to audience members for thoughtful questions. We acknowledge the work of our research assistants: Christine Kreklowitz and Russell Medved and our interviewers: Brenda Comasky, Norma Hoeppner, Rishmi Kher and Marianne Siemens.

2 . All quotes in this article are taken either from the forty-nine interview schedules completed by interviewers employed through the study or from the transcripts of taped interviews completed with ten of the forty-nine mothers.

3 . A condition of Manitoba's regulations (the jurisdiction of this study) is that subsidies are only available to parents who work or study more than twenty hours per week. A "consumer" mother is entitled to buy childcare simply on the basis of her preference; a "client" mother comes under state control and is always at potential risk of losing her subsidy if her circumstances change. It is worth pointing out that subsidy regulations are restrictive, and many parents who cannot afford full fees nevertheless do not qualify for subsidies. Only the neediest of families qualify for subsidies, and due to provincial underfunding there are not enough subsidized spaces to meet their needs.

4 . We refer in this section to directly subsidizing families using licensed childcare in Canada on the basis of income eligibility. Although childcare services are a provincial responsibility, until recently the federal Canada Assistance Plan (CAP), provided an incentive for provinces to provide subsidies to low income families by cost sharing childcare. The Liberal government's elimination of CAP and implementation of the Canada Health and Social Transfer (CHST), Bill C-76, block fund may have a far reaching effect on childcare. At the time of writing, however, it is too soon to know. Canadian families also receive financial support through the income tax system, specifically the childcare tax deduction. This support is not limited to licensed childcare and, as a tax deduction, tends to benefit higher income Canadians. For the purposes of this study, we do not consider parents who benefit from indirect tax-based support as being subsidized. *Inter alia*, we only consider mothers as "subsidized" (for the purposes of Table 1) if they receive a full subsidy from the province of Manitoba.

5 . These relatives break down as follows: 67 percent of low income mothers compared to 33 percent of middle and high income mothers were concerned. In terms of partnership status, 62 percent of mothers without partners showed concern. In contrast, less than 40 percent of mothers with partners indicated concern.

Part 5:
A Postscript:
The New Canada Child Tax Benefit

The New Canada Child Tax Benefit: Discriminating between the "Deserving" and "Undeserving" among Poor Families with Children[1]

JANE PULKINGHAM AND GORDON TERNOWETSKY

Over the last year considerable attention has been devoted to the development of new policies designed to address the growing problem of poverty among families with children. On February 18 Paul Martin presented the 1997-98 federal budget and with it the much publicized new Canada Child Tax Benefit (CCTB). Commonsense and the build-up leading to this new program of child benefits suggests that it will amount to more money for Canada's poor children. This is a noble objective, but it is not realized. Now that some of the details are out, careful examination shows that this new system is both misleading and seriously flawed as a method for enriching incomes for poor children. Federal and provincial governments are crafting an agreement that will disadvantage the poorest of poor children and their families. It will discriminate against families who receive income from provincial/territorial social assistance, in particular lone parents who rely on this form of assistance while they look after their children. It reinforces the requirement to work, even when there are not enough jobs and when existing jobs are increasingly low paid. Finally, very little, if any, "new money" from federal and provincial governments will go to poor children in the form of an income benefit.

Below we examine and critique the workings of the current Child Tax Benefit (CTB) and Working Income Supplement (WIS) and the changes announced in the 1997 federal budget. These changes will be implemented in two stages. Stage 1, beginning in July 1997, increases and restructures the WIS component of the current CTB. Stage 2, scheduled to start in July 1998, combines the enriched WIS and the CTB into one payment to form the new CCTB.

The current CTB (including the WIS) amounts to federal expenditures of $5.1 billion annually. This consists of a basic child benefit of $1,020 per child for families with incomes under $25,921. For larger families an additional $75 is paid for the third and additional children. Above the income cut-off of $25,921 benefit levels are reduced.

In addition to this basic benefit, there is also the WIS. Currently this is $500 per year per family, but in July 1997 the WIS will be changed to take into account the number of children in families. Benefits will increase from $500 per family to $605 for the first child, $405 for the second and $330 for each additional child.

In the second stage, the basic child benefit and the enriched WIS allotments will be combined to form the new CCTB. This amounts to $1,625 for the first child and $1,425 for each additional child. These CCTB payments are equivalent to the sum of the current CTB and the enriched WIS that takes effect in July 1997. The table below shows how this works by comparing the base CTB, the current and proposed July 1997 WIS benefit levels, and the value of the 1998 CCTB.

Table 1: Comparison of Current Maximum Federal Child Tax Benefits with Proposed 1998 Benefits.

	Child Tax Credit Base	Current Benefit* with WIS	July 1997 WIS Increase*	Proposed 1998 CCTB
	($)	($)	($)	($)
1 child	1,020	1,520	1,625	1,625
2 children	2,040	2,540	3,050	3,050
3 children	3,135	3,635	4,475	4,475
4 children	4,230	4,730	5,900	5,900

* Plus $213 for each child under seven when no child care expenses are claimed.

Source: Adapted from Canada, 1997a. Towards a National Child Benefit System, Ottawa: Department of Finance.

Why is this new system flawed? Consider the following. First, according to Paul Martin, the enriched CCTB represents a commitment of $850 million. There is $600 million in "new money" starting in July 1998, as well as the $250 million WIS increase announced in the 1996 budget. It is a mistake, however, to treat this $600 million as new money. Rather, it constitutes nothing more than a small repayment of funds that have been siphoned from federal transfer payments to the provinces for social assistance since the 1995-96 Liberal budget. With the elimination of the Canada Assistance Plan (CAP), which cost-shared provincial welfare assistance and services, and the introduction of the Canada Health and Social Transfer (CHST), the federal government will have reduced its welfare transfers to provinces by over $3 billion since April 1996. In addition, this $600 million in "new money" is a federal transfer that replaces money previously paid by provincial and territorial governments to families with children on public assistance. In the new agreement, provinces and territories will be able to recoup their money from the $600 million transfer. Overall, what "new money," if any, is transferred to poor families with children, remains to be seen.

A second problem is that, as a benefit directed to poor children, one would expect the announced entitlement increases to be established according to the financial needs of children. Instead, in stage 1, these are based on the work status of parents. This is a fundamental flaw. A benefit that is purportedly earmarked for poor children should not be contingent on the workforce participation of parents. In practice this means that more than 60 percent of Canada's poor children will gain nothing from this new program (Valpy 1997). What the government has done is bolster the distinction between the "deserving" and "undeserving" poor. This disenfranchising of poor children without parents in the workforce suggests that, in the view of the federal government, these children are less worthy of financial support.

In this respect stage 1, like its predecessor, is not a children's benefit. Rather it continues to be a WIS scheme, albeit enriched, for working poor families with children. On its own, a WIS has merit. However, it should not be presented as an enriched child benefit since the work status of parents, rather than the financial needs of children, is the criterion for qualifying. In addition WIS entrenches a low wage strategy. It does this in a number of ways. First, it is a part of a broader welfare strategy aimed at reducing income assistance benefits while increasing the requirement to work. Second, because of these policies, low wages become more attractive even though remuneration levels are unable to meet basic needs. In this context, WIS acts as a low wage subsidy, making low wage jobs more tolerable, enlarging the pool of people willing to take up low wage jobs and thereby intensifying a downward pressure on wages.

Another issue is that, like the earlier CTB introduced by the Mulroney Conservatives in 1992, the enriched WIS continues to penalize many of the working poor, particularly women, who work part-time and receive low or minimum wages. This occurs as the WIS begins to kick in at an annual wage of $3,750. After $10,000 the full amount of the supplement is paid up to an earned income of $20,921. With the plague of high unemployment and the spread of low wage, part-time work, income thresholds of $3,750 and $10,000 are too high as they exclude working parents who earn less. The minimum wage in many provinces for full-time, full-year work hovers around $10,000. This means that part-time workers, many of whom are women with children, will likely be excluded from receiving the full value of the WIS. The first stage of the process of enriching the existing CTB not only continues to abandon poor families in receipt of income assistance, but it also excludes the poorest of the working poor. In fact this benefit fails in its purported intent to better target families with children who are in greatest need. A further point is that the value of the CTB and the enriched WIS are not indexed to inflation. As noted by Campaign 2000 (1996b), over time this erodes the value of the benefit for poor families while it saves the federal government $160 million annually.

What about stage 2, which combines the basic child benefit of the current Child Tax Benefit (CTB) with the July 1997 restructured Work Income Supplement (WIS) to form the new CCTB? While the work status of parents is no longer the standard for receiving extra benefits, income "source" becomes the yardstick for determining whether families actually will benefit financially from the proposed CCTB. Through a new agreement (yet to be announced) the federal government will permit provinces and territories to deduct a sum equivalent to the enriched WIS component of the CCTB from income assistance payments made to families. This will fortify the distinction between the "deserving" and "undeserving" poor. The "undeserving," as in stage 1, are poor families with children who rely on public assistance as their main income source. The "deserving," those who actually benefit financially from the CCTB, are 'working poor' families with children whose primary source of income comes from employment.

The key phrase in the budget documents (one that would have been agreed to earlier in consultations with provincial social service ministers) is that "families on social assistance would receive no less overall" than they currently obtain through provincial and territorial welfare payments (Canada 1997a:6). What this means is that these families will probably gain nothing from the new CCTB. This is the case as, unlike families with equivalent net income from employment, part of the value of the federal CCTB will be deducted from families whose income derives from public assistance. The income of these families will remain pegged at the different welfare rates (and these are far below accepted standards of income adequacy) that are current in the provinces and territories.

Another key phrase states that "enriched federal benefits will enable provinces and territories to redirect" extra social assistance funds to "other programs targeted at improving work incentives and supporting children in low income families" (Canada 1997a:6; Canada 1997b:19). Two points regarding these services are warranted. First, they will be funded through the savings that accrue to the provinces and territories by deducting the enriched component of the federal CCTB from poor families with children whose "source" of income is welfare. Second, many of these services envisioned by the federal, provincial and territorial governments previously were mandated legally through the Canada Assistance Plan. With the CHST, these mandated services are lost. Now it appears that these services and benefits will be financed in part through the monies earmarked for children in poverty. It is clear, however, that most of this money will be used for low income working families. The current documentation on the CCTB says very little about services and benefits for families and children whose main source of income is public assistance (Canada 1997a:6). In effect, CAP provisions that disallowed workfare as a condition for receipt of assistance and services are now being replaced by a system of services based on a work test.

Social policy involves making choices. In considering new legislation it is important to ask: who wins, who loses and what role does the state play in reducing or reinforcing existing income and other forms of inequality. In terms of the new Canada Child Tax Benefit the answers to these questions are quite clear. At one level working poor families with children gain something, although this is a rather paltry sum. As noted by the Vanier Institute of the

Family, the new supplement to the working poor, on average, amounts to $2.13 a day. The federal government may, however, be the biggest winner as it appears to be doing something about children in poverty. Nevertheless, the analyses of the new benefit system presented above show that there is really no new money, and that additional cash components will not go to the poorest of poor children.

Today there are some 1.4 million poor children in 771,000 families (Campaign 2000 1996b). Sixty percent of these families rely primarily on income assistance, and it is these families and their children who are the real losers. There is no extra cash for them. In this respect, the CCTB ends up reinforcing the impoverishment of the poorest of poor children in this country.

The government's approach to enriching child benefits has a number of key problems. First, it ignores the reality that, in today's new economy, there are not enough jobs to go around and the jobs that do exist are increasingly low paid. Second, caring for children (the reason many single parents are on income assistance) is in itself a valuable contribution that is undervalued. This is a policy that clearly discriminates against lone parents who have no alternative way of supporting themselves while caring for their children full-time. Despite this, the government has chosen to pursue a policy that suggests that parents and children from working poor families (stage 1), whose main source of income comes from employment (stage 2) are more "deserving" of assistance than children raised in families that are primarily dependent on welfare incomes for economic survival. In this way, the federal Liberals continue their neoliberal agenda where their benevolence and concern for Canada's poorest children are more apparent than real.

Note

1.   We would like to thank David Hay for his comments and suggestions on an earlier draft of this article.

Bibliography

Abbott, P., and C. Wallace. 1992. *The Family and the New Right*. London: Pluto Press.

Aboriginal Community Panel. 1992. *Liberating Our Children, Liberating Our Nations*. Report of the Aboriginal Committee Community Panel Family and Children's Services Legislation Review in British Columbia. Vancouver: British Columbia Social Services.

Adkin, L.E. 1992. "Counter-Hegemony and Environmental Politics in Canada." In W.K. Carroll (ed.), *Organizing Dissent, Contemporary Social Movements in Theory and Practice*. Toronto: Garamond Press.

Aldridge, M. 1990. "Social Work and the News Media: A Hopeless Case?" *British Journal of Social Work* 20:611-25.

Allen, D.W. 1995. "Some Comments Regarding Divorce, Lone Mothers, and Children." In M.D. Dooley, R. Finnie, S.A. Phipps, and N. Naylor (eds.), *Family Matters: New Policies for Divorce, Lone Mothers, and Child Poverty*. Toronto: C.D. Howe Institute.

Allen, R.C., and G. Rosenbluth. 1992. *False Promises: The Failure of Conservative Economics*. Vancouver: New Star Books.

Angus, M. 1991. *And the Last Shall Be First: Native Policy in an Era of Cutbacks*. Toronto: NC Press.

Armitage, A. 1993a. "Family and Child Welfare in First Nations Communities." In B. Wharf (ed.), *Rethinking Child Welfare in Canada*. Toronto: McClelland and Stewart.

_____. 1993b. "The Policy and Legislative Context." In B. Wharf (ed.), *Rethinking Child Welfare in Canada*. Toronto: McClelland and Stewart.

Aucoin, P., and H. Bakvis. 1988. *The Centralization–Decentralization Conundrum: Organization and Management in the Canadian Government*. Halifax: Institute for Research on Public Policy.

Bach, M., and M. Rioux. 1996. "Social Policy, Devolution and Disability: Back to Notions of the Worthy Poor." In J. Pulkingham and G. Ternowetsky (eds.), *Remaking Canadian Social Policy: Social Security in the Late 1990s*. Halifax: Fernwood.

Baines, C., P. Evans, and S. Neysmith, eds. 1991. *Women's Caring: Feminist Perspectives on Social Welfare*. Toronto: McClelland and Stewart.

Baker, G., and J. Warnyca, 1996. "Family Nights at Day Care." *Interaction* 9(4): 33-36.

Baker, M. 1990. *Families: Changing Trends in Canada*. Toronto: McGraw-Hill Ryerson.

_____. (ed.). 1994. *Canada's Changing Families: Challenges to Public Policy*. Ottawa: Vanier Institute of the Family.

_____. 1995a. *Canadian Family Policies: Cross-National Comparisons*. Toronto: University of Toronto Press.

_____. 1995b. "Women, Family Policies and the Moral Right." Prepared for the annual meetings of the Canadian Sociology and Anthropology Association, Montreal: June 1995.

_____. 1997. "Advocacy, Political Alliances and the Implementation of Family Policies." In J. Pulkingham and G. Ternowetsky (eds.), *Child and Family Policies: Struggles, Strategies and Options*. Halifax: Fernwood.

Baker, M., and M.A. Robeson. 1986. "Trade Union Reactions to Women Workers and Their Concerns." In K. Lundy and B. Warme (eds.), *Work in the Canadian Context*. Second edition. Toronto: Butterworths.

Bala, N. 1991. "An Introduction to Child Protection Problems." In N. Bala, J. P. Hornick and R. Vogl (eds.), *Canadian Child Welfare Law*. Toronto: Thompson Educational Publishing.

Balbo, L. 1987. "Crazy Quilts: Rethinking the Welfare State Debate from a Woman's Point of View." In A. Sassoon (ed.), *Women and the State: The Shifting Boundaries of Public and Private*. London: Hutchinson.

Banting, K. 1985. "Universality and the Development of the Welfare State." In A. Green and N. Olewiler (eds.), *Report of the Forum on Universality and Social Policies in the 1990s*. Kingston: Queen's University Press.

_____ . 1987. *The Welfare State and Canadian Federalism*. Kingston and Montreal: McGill-Queen's University Press.

Banting, K.G., C. M. Beach, and G. Betcherman. 1995. "Polarization and Social Policy Reform: Evidence and Issues." In K.G. Banting and C.M. Beach (eds.), *Labour Market Polarization and Social Policy Reform*. Kingston: School of Policy Studies, Queen's University.

Barlow, M. 1996. "Budget Blight." *The Canadian Forum* 75(849):9.

Barnhorst, D., and B. Walter. 1991. "Child Protection Legislation in Canada." In N. Bala, J.P. Hornick and R. Vogl (eds.), *Canadian Child Welfare Law*. Toronto: Thompson Educational Publishing.

Barthes, R. 1988. "Textual Analysis: Poe's 'Valdemar.'" *Modern Criticism and Theory*. Longman: London.

Battle, K. 1995. *Government Fights Growing Gap Between Rich and Poor*. Ottawa: Caledon Institute of Social Policy.

Battle, K., and L. Muszynski. 1995. *One Way to Fight Child Poverty*. Ottawa: Caledon Institute of Social Policy.

Battle, K., and S. Torjman. 1993. *Federal Social Programs: Setting the Record Straight*. Ottawa: Caledon Institute of Social Policy.

_____ . 1995. *How Finance Re-Formed Social Policy*. Ottawa: Caledon Institute of Social Policy.

_____ . 1996. "Desperately Seeking Substance: A Commentary on the Social Security Review." In J. Pulkingham and G. Ternowetsky (eds.), *Remaking Canadian Social Policy: Social Security in the Late 1990s*. Halifax: Fernwood.

Baxter, S. 1993. *A Child Is Not a Toy: Voices of Children in Poverty*. Vancouver: New Star Books.

BC Campaign 2000. 1995. *Invest in Our Future, Invest in Canadian Children: Report Card 1995*. Vancouver: BC Campaign 2000.

_____ . 1996a. *Child Poverty Community Action Kit*. Vancouver: BC Campaign 2000.

_____ . 1996b. *Child Poverty in British Columbia: Report Card 1996*. Vancouver: BC Campaign 2000.

_____ . 1996c. *Community Actions on Child Poverty throughout BC for November 18, 1996*. Vancouver: BC Campaign 2000.

_____ . 1996d. *170,000 BC Children Live in Poverty*. News Release. Vancouver: BC Campaign 2000.

BDO Ward Mallette. 1991. *Critique of a Proposed Funding Formula for Child and Family Services*. Unpublished report for Manitoba First Nations Child and Family Services Agencies. Winnipeg: Manitoba.

Bell, S., and H. Munro. 1996. "Suffer the Children: The BC Ombudsman for Children says 170,000 Youngsters are Living in Poverty and Welfare Cuts are Making it Worse."

Vancouver Sun, November 19, B1-2.

Bellemare, D. 1993. "The History of Economic Insecurity." In D. Ross et al. (eds.), *Family Security in Insecure Times: National Forum on Family Security.* Ottawa: Canadian Council on Social Development.

Bennett, T. 1982. "Media, 'Reality,' Signification." In M. Gurevitch, T. Bennett, J. Curran and J. Woliacott (eds.), *Culture, Society and the Media.* New York: Methuen.

Biggs, M. 1996. *Building Blocks for Canada's New Social Union.* Working Paper No. F02. Ottawa: Canadian Policy Research Networks Inc.

Birchall, C. 1996. "Open Letter to Paul Martin re: Budget 1996." Canadian Council on Social Development brief. Ottawa: CCSD.

Blau, J. 1989. "Theories of the Welfare State." *Social Service Review* 63(1):26-38.

Boldt, M. 1993. *Surviving as Indians: The Challenge of Self-Government.* Toronto: University of Toronto Press.

Bookman, A. 1991. "Parenting Without Poverty: The Case for Funded Parental Leave." In J.S. Hyde and M.J. Essex (eds.), *Parental Leave and Child Care.* Philadelphia: Temple University Press.

Boreham, P., and H. Compston. 1992. "Labour Movement Organization and Political Intervention: The Politics of Unemployment in the OECD Countries, 1974-1986." *European Journal of Political Research* 22(August):143-70.

Bourgeault, R. 1983. "The Indian, the Métis and the Fur Trade. Classism, Sexism and Racism in the Transition from 'Communism' to 'Capitalism.'" *Studies in Political Economy* 12:45-86.

Brant, C. 1990. "Native Ethics and Rules of Behaviour." *Canadian Journal of Psychiatry* 35(6):534-39.

Bravo, E. 1991. "Family Leave: The Need for a New Minimum Standard." In J.S. Hyde and M.J. Essex (eds.), *Parental Leave and Child Care.* Philadelphia: Temple University Press.

Briskin, L., and L. Yanz. 1985. *Union Sisters.* Second edition. Toronto: Women's Press.

British Columbia. 1979. *Social Workers Act.* Victoria: Queen's Printer.

_____. 1994. *Child, Family and Community Service Act.* Victoria: Queen's Printer.

Brodie, J. 1995. *Politics on the Margins: Restructuring and the Canadian Women's Movement.* Halifax: Fernwood.

Brodie, J., and J. Jenson. 1988. *Crisis, Challenge and Change.* Ottawa: Carleton University Press.

Brownlee, K., and S. Taylor. 1995. "CASW Code of Ethics and Non-Sexual Dual Relationships: The Need for Clarification." *The Social Worker* 63(3):133-36.

Buchbinder, H. 1979. "The Just Society Movement." In B. Wharf (ed.), *Community Work in Canada.* Toronto: McClelland and Stewart.

Burford, G., and J. Pennell. 1995. "Family Group Decision Making: An Innovation in Child and Family Welfare." In J. Hudson and B. Galaway (eds.), *Child Welfare in Canada: Research and Policy Implications.* Toronto: Thompson Educational Publishing.

Cage, R. 1988. "Criminal Investigation of Sexual Abuse Cases." In S.M. Sgroi (ed.), *Vulnerable Populations. Volume I: Evaluation and Treatment of Sexually Abused Children and Adult Survivors.* Toronto: Lexington Books, D.C. Heath and Company.

Caledon Institute of Social Policy. 1996. *Sustainable Social Policy and Community Capital.* Ottawa: Caledon Institute of Social Policy and the Canada Mortgage and Housing Corporation.

Callahan, M. 1993a. "The Administrative and Practice Context: Perspectives from the Front-Line." In B. Wharf (ed.), *Rethinking Child Welfare in Canada*. Toronto: McClelland and Stewart.

_____. 1993b. "Feminist Approaches: Women Recreate Child Welfare." In B. Wharf (ed.), *Rethinking Child Welfare in Canada*. Toronto: McClelland and Stewart.

_____. 1994. "Stereotypes of Women in Child Welfare." Unpublished doctoral dissertation. Bristol: University of Bristol, School of Social Planning and Social Administration.

Callahan, M., and K. Callahan. 1997. "Victims and Villains: Scandals, the Press and Policy Making in Child Welfare." In J. Pulkingham and G. Ternowetsky (eds.), *Child and Family Policies: Struggles, Strategies and Options*. Halifax: Fernwood.

Callender, C. 1996. Personal communication. Staff person, CD Howe Institute.

Cammaert, L.A. 1988. "Nonoffending Mothers: A New Conceptualization." In L.E.A. Walker (ed.), *Handbook on Sexual Abuse of Children*. New York: Springer Publishing Company.

Campaign 2000. 1992. *Child Poverty in Canada: Report Card 1992*. Toronto: Campaign 2000.

_____. 1993. *Child Poverty in Canada: Report Card 1993*. Toronto: Campaign 2000.

_____. 1994a. *Countdown 94: Campaign 2000 Child Poverty Indicator Report*. Ottawa: Canadian Council on Social Development.

_____. 1994b. *Child Poverty in Canada: Report Card 1994*. Toronto: Campaign 2000.

_____. 1994c. *Investing in the Next Generation: Policy Perspectives on Children and Nationhood*. Toronto: Campaign 2000.

_____. 1995a. *Countdown*. Toronto: Campaign 2000.

_____. 1995b. *Child Poverty in Canada: Report Card 1995*. Toronto: Campaign 2000.

_____. 1996a. *Crossroads for Canada: A Time to Invest in Children and Families*. Discussion Paper. November. Toronto: Campaign 2000.

_____. 1996b. *Child Poverty in Canada: Report Card 1996*. Toronto: Campaign 2000.

Campaign 2000. 1997. *Child Poverty in Canada: Report Card 1996*. Toronto: Ontario.

Campbell, M. 1995. "Wonks." *The Globe and Mail,* December 2, D1.

Canada. 1985. *Notes on Welfare Services Under the Canada Assistance Plan*. Ottawa: Minister of National Health and Welfare.

_____. 1992. *The Child Benefit. A White Paper on Canada's New Integrated Child Tax Benefit*. Ottawa: Minister of Supply and Services.

_____. 1993. *Towards 2000: Eliminating Child Poverty*. Report of the Standing Committee on Health and Welfare, Social Affairs, Seniors and the Status of Women. Ottawa: Queen's Printer.

_____. 1994. *Income Security for Children: A Supplementary Paper*. Ottawa: Minister of Supply and Services.

_____. 1995. *Budget Plan*. Ottawa: Department of Finance.

_____. 1997a. *Towards a National Child Benefit System*. Ottawa: Department of Finance.

_____. 1997b. *Working Together Towards a National Child Benefit*. Ottawa: Department of Finance.

Canada, Government of. 1992. *Brighter Futures. Canada's Action Plan for Children*. Ottawa: Minister of Supply and Services.

Canada, House of Commons. 1987. *Sharing Our Responsibility*. Report of the Special Committee on Child Care (Chaired by Shirley Martin, MP). March. Ottawa: Supply and Services.

_____. 1989. *Commons Debate*. November 24: 6173-6228. Ottawa: House of Commons.

_____. 1991. *Canada's Children. Investing in the Future*. Report of the Standing Committee on Health and Welfare, Social Affairs, Seniors and the Status of Women (Sub-Committee on Poverty, Chaired by Barbara Greene, MP). Ottawa: House of Commons.

Canada, Senate. 1989. *Child Poverty and Adult Social Problems*. Report of the Standing Senate Committee on Social Affairs, Science and Technology (Chaired by Senators Lorna Marsden and Brenda Robertson). Ottawa: The Senate.

_____. 1991. *Children in Poverty: Toward a Better Future*. Report of the Standing Senate Committee on Social Affairs, Science and Technology (Chaired by Senators Lorna Marsden and Brenda Robertson). Ottawa: The Senate.

Canadian Child Welfare Association, Canadian Council on Children and Youth, Canadian Council on Social Development, Canadian Institute of Child Health, Child Poverty Action Group, Family Service Canada, Vanier Institute of the Family. 1988. *A Choice of Futures: Canada's Commitment to Its Children*. Ottawa: Canadian Council on Social Development.

Canadian Council on Social Development (CCSD). 1996a. "Children and the 1996 Federal Budget." Backgrounder. Ottawa: CCSD.

_____. 1996b. "Maintaining a National Social Safety Net: Recommendations on the Canada Health and Social Transfer." Position statement. Ottawa: CCSD.

_____. 1996c. *Social Policy Beyond the Budget*. Ottawa: CCSD.

Canadian Labour Congress. 1995. "Federal Budget 1995: Canadian Labour Congress Analysis." Unpublished brief. February 27.

Cannata, R. 1994. "Two faces of child killer: Sweet, then bitter: Vaudreuil's personality dissected." *The Vancouver Sun,* September 14, B3.

Cardozo, A. 1995. "Index on Cuts to Interest Groups." *The Canadian Forum* 74(840):48.

Carroll, W.K., (ed.). 1992. *Organizing Dissent.* Toronto: Garamond Press.

Carter, B. 1990. "But You Should Have Known: Child Sexual Abuse and the Non-Offending Mother." Unpublished doctoral dissertation. Toronto: University of Toronto.

_____. 1995. *Case Management Review and Analysis of Child Protection Services in the Province of British Columbia: 1986-1994*. A report prepared for the Gove Inquiry into Child Protection. Vancouver: B.C. Government Publications.

Cassidy, F. 1990. "Aboriginal Governments in Canada: An Emerging Field of Study." *Canadian Journal of Political Science* 23(1):73–90.

CD Howe Institute. 1996. *1995 Annual Report.* Toronto: CD Howe Institute.

Cheal, D. 1991. *Family Finances: Money Management in Breadwinner/Homemaker Families, Dual Earner Families, and Dual Career Families*. Winnipeg Area Study Research Reports, No. 38. Winnipeg: University of Manitoba, Department of Sociology.

Chibnall, S. 1977. *Law and Order News: An Analysis of Crime Reporting in the British Press.* London: Tavistock.

Child Poverty Action Group. 1986. *A Fair Chance For All Children: The Declaration on Child Poverty.* Toronto: Child Poverty Action Group.

_____. 1994. *A Federal Agenda for the Economic Security of Families, Submission to the Standing Committee on Human Resources Development.* Toronto: Child Poverty Action Group.

Child Poverty Action Group, Citizens for Public Justice and SOCIAL PLANNING COUN-CIL OF METROPOLITAN TORONTO. 1994. *Paying for Canada: Perspectives on Public Finance and National Programs.* Toronto: Social Planning Council of Metropolitan Toronto.

Child Poverty Action Group, Family Service Association of Metropolitan Toronto and Social Planning Council of Metropolitan Toronto. 1994a. *The Outsiders: A Report on the Prospects for Young Families in Metro Toronto.* Toronto: Family Service Association.

_____ . 1994b. *Voices of Young Families.* Toronto: Family Service Association.

_____ . 1995. *Young Families in Metro Toronto: A Policy Blueprint for Action.* Toronto: Family Service Association.

Childcare Resource and Research Unit. 1993. *Child Care in Canada.* Toronto: University of Toronto, Childcare Resource and Research Unit, Centre for Urban Studies.

Christian, W. 1994. Personal interview. October 25.

City of Vancouver. 1994. *Distribution of Poverty in Vancouver.* Vancouver: City of Vancouver, Social Planning Department.

Clark, C. 1995. "Work and Welfare: Looking at Both Sides of the Equation." *Perception* 19(1):21-24.

Clarkson, L., V. Morrissette, and G. Regallet. 1992. *Our Responsibility to the Seventh Generation: Indigenous People and Sustainable Development.* Winnipeg: International Institute of Sustainable Development.

Clement, W., and J. Myles. 1994. *Relations of Ruling.* Montreal and Kingston: McGill-Queen's University Press.

Cohen, J. 1985. "Strategy or Identity: New Theoretical Paradigms and Contemporary Social Movements." *Social Research* 52(4):663-716.

Cohen, J.L., and A. Arato. 1992. *Civil Society and Political Theory.* Cambridge: MIT Press.

Colwell, M.A.C. 1993. *Private Foundations and Public Policy.* New York: Garland Publishing.

Contratto, S. 1986. "Child Abuse and the Politics of Care." *Journal of Education* 168(3):70-79.

Coontz, S. 1992. *The Way We Never Were: American Families and the Nostalgia Trip.* New York: Basic.

Coopers and Lybrand Consulting Group. 1987. *An Assessment of Services Delivered Under the Canada–Manitoba Indian Child Welfare Agreement.* Winnipeg: Coopers and Lybrand Consulting Group.

Courchene, T. 1986. *Social Policy in the 1990s: Agenda for Reform.* Scarborough: Prentice-Hall.

_____ . 1994. *Social Canada in the Millennium.* Toronto: CD Howe Institute.

Crate, G. 1992. "Grassroots and Power." *The Winnipeg Sun,* May 8, 23.

Crompton, S. 1996. "Transfer Payments to Families With Children." *Perspectives on Labour and Income* 8(Autumn):42-48.

Dale, J., and P. Foster. 1986. *Feminists and State Welfare.* Boston: Routledge and Kegan Paul.

David, M. 1991. "Putting on an Act for Children?" In M. Maclean and D. Groves (eds.), *Women's Issues in Social Policy.* New York: Routledge.

Department of Finance. 1984. *A New Direction for Canada: An Agenda for Economic Renewal.* Ottawa: Minister of Supply and Services.

_____ . 1994a. *Agenda: Jobs and Growth. A New Framework for Economic Policy.* Ottawa: Department of Finance.

_____ . 1994b. *Agenda, Jobs and Growth. Creating a Healthy Fiscal Climate.* Ottawa: Department of Finance.

_____ . 1995. *Budget Speech.* Ottawa: Minister of Supply and Services.

_____ . 1996a. "Government Proposes New Seniors Benefit." News Release. Ottawa: Department of Finance.

_____ . 1996b. *Canada Health and Social Transfer.* Backgounder. Ottawa: Department of Finance.

_____ . 1996c. *Canada Health and Social Transfer: New Five Year Funding Arrangement.* Ottawa: Department of Finance.

Department of Supply and Services. 1996. *The 1996 Federal Budget.* Ottawa: Department of Supply and Services.

Doherty, G. 1991. *Quality Matters in Child Care.* Huntsville, Ontario: Jesmond Publishing.

Doyal, L., and I. Gough. 1991. *A Theory of Human Need.* New York: Guilford.

Drover, G., and P. Kerans (eds.). 1993. *New Approaches to Welfare Theory.* Aldershot, England: Edward Elgar.

Duffy, A., and N. Pupo. 1992. *Part-time Paradox. Connecting Gender, Work and Family.* Toronto: McClelland and Stewart.

Dumont, R. 1988. "Culturally Selective Perceptions in Child Welfare Decisions." *The Social Worker* 56(4):149-52. Durst, D., J. McDonald, and C. Rich. 1995. "Aboriginal Government of Child Welfare Services: Hobson's Choice?" In J. Hudson and B. Galaway (eds.), *Child Welfare in Canada: Research and Policy Implications.* Toronto: Thompson Educational Publishing.

Economic Council of Canada. 1990. *Good Jobs, Bad Jobs.* Ottawa: Department of Supply and Services.

Ecumenical Coalition for Economic Justice (ECEJ). 1993. *Reweaving Canada's Social Programs: From Shredded Safety Net to Social Solidarity.* Toronto: Our Times.

_____ . 1996. *Promises to Keep, Miles to Go: An Examination of Canada's Record in the International Year for the Eradication of Poverty (1996).* Toronto: Ecumenical Coalition for Economic Justice.

Edelman, M. 1988. *Constructing the Political Spectacle.* Chicago: University of Chicago Press.

Eichler, M. 1988a. *Nonsexist Research Methods: A Practical Guide.* Boston: Allen and Unwin.

_____ . 1988b. *Families in Canada Today: Recent Changes and Their Policy Consequences.* Toronto: Gage.

_____ . 1988c. *Fifty Questions: Problems and Issues in Developing Policies for Canadian Families.* Family Policy Series, Publication No. 1. Ottawa: Canadian Centre for Policy Alternatives.

Eisenstein, Z. 1981. *The Radical Future of Liberal Feminism.* New York: Longman.

Eisler, D. 1996. "Prairie Time Bomb." *Maclean's* 109(46):18-19.

Ekos Research Associates Inc. 1995. *Rethinking Government '94.* Ottawa: Ekos Research Associates Inc.

Employment and Immigration Canada. 1994. *Unemployment Insurance Account: Forecasts from 1994 to 1998.* Ottawa: Employment and Immigration Canada.

End Legislated Poverty. 1996. *Government Progress Report.* Vancouver: End Legislated Poverty.

Epp, J. 1986. "Achieving Health for All: A Framework for Health Promotion." *Canadian Journal of Public Health* 77(6):393-430.

Esping-Andersen, G. 1985. *Politics Against Markets: The Social Democratic Road to Power.* Cambridge: University of Harvard Press.

_____. 1990. *The Three Worlds of Welfare Capitalism.* Princeton: Princeton University Press.

Evans, P. 1996. "Single Mothers and Ontario's Welfare Policy: Restructuring the Debate." In J. Brodie (ed.), *Women and Canadian Public Policy.* Toronto: Harcourt Brace and Company, Canada.

Everson, M., W. Hunter, D. Runyon, G. Edelson, and M. Coulter. 1989. "Maternal Support Following Disclosure of Incest." *American Journal of Orthopsychiatry* 59(2):197-207.

Faller, K. 1988. "The Myth of the 'Collusive Mother.'" *Journal of Interpersonal Violence* 3(2):190-96.

Faludi, S. 1991. *Backlash.* New York: Crown Publishers.

Federal, Provincial and Territorial Advisory Committee on Population Health. 1994. *Strategies for Population Health: Investing in the Health of Canadians.* Ottawa: Minister of Supply and Services.

_____. 1996. *Report on the Health of Canadians.* Ottawa: Minister of Supply and Services.

Ferguson, E. 1991. "The Child-Care Crisis: The Realities of Women's Caring." In C. Baines, P. Evans and S. Neysmith (eds.), *Women's Caring: Feminist Perspectives on Social Welfare.* Toronto: McClelland and Stewart.

_____. 1992. "Public or Private? Profit or Non-Profit? Reasons for the Auspice Preference of a Sample of Daycare Consumers in Ontario." Unpublished doctoral dissertation. Toronto, University of Toronto, Faculty of Social Work.

Findlay, S. 1993. "Problematizing Privilege: Another Look at Representation." In L. Carty (ed.), *And Still We Rise: Feminist Political Mobilizing in Contemporary Canada.* Toronto: Women's Press.

Finkelhor, D. 1984. *Child Sexual Abuse: New Theory and Research.* New York: The Free Press.

First Call. 1996. *An Overview of Child and Youth Issues in British Columbia.* Vancouver: First Call, BC Child and Youth Advocacy Coalition.

First Nations Child and Family Task Force. 1993. *Children First: Our Responsibility.* Winnipeg: Manitoba Family Services.

Flynn, J. 1992. *Social Agency Policy.* Second edition. Chicago: Nelson-Hall.

Forget, C., R. Bennet, M. Morgan, Jack Munro, G. Saucier, and F. Soboda. 1986. *Commission of Inquiry on Unemployment Insurance.* Ottawa: Minister of Supply and Services.

Foucault, M. 1980. *Power/Knowledge.* Colin Gordon (ed.), C. Gordon, L. Marshall, J. Mepham, and K. Soper (trans.). New York: Pantheon Books.

Franklin, B., and N. Parton. 1991. *Social Work, the Media and Public Relations.* London: Routledge.

Fraser, N. 1989. "Struggle Over Needs: Outline of a Socialist-Feminist Critical Theory of Late Capitalist Political Culture." In N. Fraser (ed.), *Unruly Practices.* Minneapolis: University of Minnesota Press.

Fraser, N., and L. Gordon. 1994. "A Genealogy of Dependency: Tracing a Keyword of the U.S. Welfare State." *Signs* 19(21):309-36.

Fraser Institute. 1995. *1994 Annual Report.* Vancouver: Fraser Institute.

_____ . 1996. *1995 Annual Report.* Vancouver: Fraser Institute.

Freiler, C. 1995. "Block funding adds to child poverty levels." *Winnipeg Free Press,* March 8, A7.

Frideres, J.S. 1988. *Native People in Canada: Contemporary Conflicts.* Scarborough: Prentice-Hall.

Friendly, M. 1994. *Child Care Policy in Canada: Putting the Pieces Together.* Don Mills: Addison-Wesley.

Fry, A. 1991. "Reporting Social Work: A View From the Newsroom." In B. Franklin and N. Parton (eds.), *Social Work, the Media and Public Relations.* London: Routledge.

Gadd, J. 1996a. "Radical Steps Urged to End Child Poverty." *The Globe and Mail,* November 26, A3.

_____. 1996b. "Romanow Says Cuts Affecting Children: Premier Joins Call to Restore Services." *The Globe and Mail,* November 28, A4.

Garrett, P., D. Wenk, and S. Lubeck. 1990. "Working Around Childbirth: Comparative and Empirical Perspectives on Parental Leave Policy." *Child Welfare* 69(5):401-13.

Gavey, N., J. Florence, S. Pezaro, and J. Tan. 1990. "Mother-Blaming, the Perfect Alibi: Family Therapy and the Mothers of Incest Survivors." *Journal of Feminist Family Therapy* 2(1):1-25.

Giesbrecht, D. 1992. *Report of the Fatality Inquiries Act Respecting the Death of Lester Norman Desjarlais.* Winnipeg: Queen's Printer.

Glaser, D., and S. Frosh. 1993. *Child Sexual Abuse.* Second edition. Toronto: University of Toronto Press.

Globe and Mail. 1996a. "Residents Among the World's Healthiest." *The Globe and Mail,* March 5, A4.

_____. 1996b. "Child Poverty: Facing the Choices." Editorial. *The Globe and Mail,* November 28, A20.

_____. 1996c. "Who's Hot—Who's Not." *The Globe and Mail,* November 30, A4.

_____. 1996d. "It's All In The Delivery." *The Globe and Mail,* November 30, A4.

Gordon, I.J., P.P. Olmstead, R.I. Rubin, and J.H. True. 1979. "How Has Follow Through Promoted Parent Involvement?" *Young Children* 34(5):49-53.

Gove Inquiry into Child Protection. 1994a. Transcripts. September 13:1733-34.

_____ . 1994b. Transcripts. September 27:227.

Gove, T. 1995. *Report of the Gove Inquiry into Child Protection in British Columbia.* Vancouver: B.C. Government Publications.

Gray-Withers, D. 1997. "Decentralized Social Services and Self-Government: Challenges for First Nations." In J. Pulkingham and G. Ternowetsky (eds.), *Child and Family Policies: Struggles, Strategies and Options.* Halifax: Fernwood.

Green, D.A., and C.W. Riddell. 1993. "The Economic Effects of Unemployment Insurance in Canada: An Empirical Analysis of UI Disentitlement." *Journal of Labor Economics* 11(1)(2):S96-S147.

Greenspon, E. 1996a. "Dingwall Takes Aim at Child Poverty." *The Globe and Mail,* November 26, A1, 3.

_____. 1996b. "Child Poverty Relief Not Ready Yet." *The Globe and Mail,* November 27, A6.

_____. 1996c. "Fight Against Child Poverty Unites Ottawa, Provinces: Joint National Benefit Program Supported in Principle." *The Globe and Mail,* November 28, A4.

Guest, D. 1980. *The Emergence of Social Security in Canada.* Vancouver: University of British Columbia Press.

Gunderson, M., L. Muszynski, and J. Keck. 1990. *Women and Labour Market Poverty.* Ottawa: Canadian Advisory Council on the Status of Women.

Haas, L. 1991. "Equal Parenthood and Social Policy: Lessons from a Study of Parental Leave in Sweden." In J.S. Hyde and M.J. Essex (eds.), *Parental Leave and Child Care.* Philadelphia: Temple University Press.

Habermas, J. 1996. *Between Facts and Norms.* Translated by William Rehg. Cambridge: MIT Press.

Hachey, L., and M. Grenier. 1992. "The Attribution of Causality in Lepine Murder News." In Grenier, M. (ed.), *Critical Studies of Canadian Mass Media.* Toronto: Butterworths.

Haddow, R. 1990. "The Poverty Policy Community in Canada's Liberal Welfare State." In William D. Coleman and Grace Skogstad (eds.), *Policy Communities and Public Policy in Canada: A Structural Approach.* Mississauga: Copp Clark Pitman.

_____. 1993. *Poverty Reform in Canada, 1958-1978.* Montreal and Kingston: McGill-Queen's University Press.

Hamilton, A., and M. Sinclair. 1991. *Volume 1: The Justice System and Aboriginal People.* Report of the Aboriginal Justice Inquiry. Winnipeg: Queen's Printer.

Handler, E. 1973. "The Expectation of Daycare Parents." *The Social Service Review* 47(3):266-67.

Hargrove, B. 1996. "Whose unemployment-insurance surplus is it, anyway?" *The Globe and Mail,* March 18, A17.

Hay, D.I. 1993a. "Campaign 2000: Putting an End to Child Poverty." *SPARC News: Community Affairs in British Columbia* 10(1):16-17.

_____. 1993b. "Does Money Buy Health? An Empirical Investigation of the Relationship Between Income and Health." Vancouver: Social Planning and Research Council of BC.

_____. 1994. "Social Status and Health Status: Does Money Buy Health?" In B.S. Bolaria and R. Bolaria (eds.), *Racial Minorities, Medicine and Health.* Halifax: Fernwood.

_____. 1995a. "What's the Bottom Line" *SPARC News: Community Affairs in British Columbia* 12(1):inside front cover.

_____. 1995b. "MPs Get Failing Report Card on Child Poverty." *SPARC News: Community Affairs in British Columbia* 12(2):3-4.

_____. 1996. "170,000 BC Children Living in Poverty." *SPARC News: Community Affairs in British Columbia* 13(2):8-9.

_____. 1997. "Campaign 2000: Family and Child Poverty in Canada." In J. Pulkingham and G. Ternowetsky (eds.), *Child and Family Policies: Struggles, Strategies and Options.* Halifax: Fernwood.

Hayes, C., J.L. Palmer, and M.J. Zaslow, (eds.). 1990. *Who Cares for America's Children. Child Care Policy for the 1990s.* Washington, DC.: National Academy Press.

Haysom, I. 1994. "Editorial." *The Vancouver Sun,* November 19, A24.

Herman, E., and N. Chomsky. 1988. *Manufacturing Consent: The Political Economy of the Mass Media.* New York: Pantheon Books.

Hess, M. 1992. *The Canadian Fact Book on Income Security Programs.* Ottawa: Canadian Council on Social Development.

_____. 1993. *An Overview of Canadian Social Policy.* Ottawa: Canadian Council on Social Development.

Honneth, A. 1991. *The Critique of Power.* Cambridge: MIT Press.

Hooper, C. 1992. *Mothers Surviving Child Sexual Abuse*. New York: Tavistock/ Routledge.

Horejsi, C., J. Bertsche, S. Francetich, B. Collins, and R. Francetich. 1987. "Protocols in Child Welfare: An Example." *Child Welfare* 66(5):423-31.

Horry, I., F. Palda, and M. Walker. 1995. *Tax Facts 9*. Vancouver: Fraser Institute.

Hoschild, A. 1983. *The Managed Heart: Commercialization of Human Feeling*. Berkeley: University of California.

Hubka, D.S. 1992. "Reporting on Child Poverty: The Efforts of Campaign 2000." *Perception* 16(4) Fall:17-22.

Hudson, P., and B. McKenzie. 1981. "Child Welfare and Native People: The Extension of Colonialism." *The Social Worker* 49(2):63-66, 87-88.

_____. 1984. *Evaluation of Dakota Ojibway Child and Family Services*. Ottawa: Indian and Northern Affairs Canada.

Hudson, P., and S. Taylor-Henley. 1987a. *Agreement and Disagreement: An Evaluation of the Canada-Manitoba Indian Child Welfare Agreement*. Winnipeg: University of Manitoba, School of Social Work.

_____. 1987b. *Indian Provincial Relationships in Social Welfare: Northern Issues and Future Options* (Child and Family Services Research Group Series #0476). Winnipeg: University of Manitoba, School of Social Work.

_____. 1993. "Linking Social and Political Developments in First Nation Communities." In A.M. MaWhinney (ed.), *Rebirth: Political, Economic and Social Development in First Nations*. Sudbury: Laurentian University, Institute of Northern Ontario Research and Development.

_____. 1995. "First Nations Child and Family Services, 1982-1992: Facing the Realities." *Canadian Social Work Review* 12(Winter):72-84.

Human Resources Development Canada (HRDC). 1994a. *Agenda: Jobs and Growth: Improving Social Security in Canada*. Ottawa: Supply and Services.

_____. 1994b. *Guaranteed Annual Income: A Supplementary Paper*. Ottawa: Minister of Supply and Services.

_____. 1994c. *Inventory of Income Security Programs in Canada*. Ottawa: Minister of Supply and Services.

_____. 1996a. *Employment Insurance. Impacts of Reform*. Submisssion to the House of Commons Standing Committee on Human Resources Development. January 23. Ottawa: HRDC.

_____. 1996b. "Why Has the Child Poverty Rate Failed to Fall?" *Applied Research Bulletin* 2(2):1-3.

_____. 1996c. "Labour Market Polarization . . . What's Going On?" *Applied Research Bulletin* 2(2):5-7.

Humphreys, C. 1994. "Counteracting Mother-Blaming Among Child Sexual Abuse Service Providers: An Experiential Workshop." *Journal of Feminist Family Therapy* 6(1):49-65.

Hutchison, E. 1992. "Child Welfare as a Woman's Issue." *Families in Society: The Journal of Contemporary Human Services* 73(2):67-78.

Indian and Northern Affairs Canada. 1989. *Indian and Child and Family Services Management Regime Discussion Paper*. Ottawa: INAC.

Indigenous Women's Collective of Manitoba Inc. 1993. *Report on the Indigenous Women's Perspective in Manitoba for the Royal Commission on Aboriginal Peoples*. Submitted by C. McKay. Winnipeg: Indigenous Women's Collective of Manitoba Inc.

_____. 1994. *Report of the Discussion on the Inherent Right to Self-Government.* Submitted by E.J. Courchene. Winnipeg: Indigenous Women's Collective of Manitoba Inc.

International Labour Organization. 1995. *World Employment 1995.* Geneva: International Labour Organization.

Ip, G. 1996. "Why Productivity Goes Up and People Go Down." *The Globe and Mail,* November 30, D1-2.

Jackson, S. 1995. "Looking After Children Better: An Interactive Model for Research and Practice." In J. Hudson and B. Galaway (eds.), *Child Welfare in Canada: Research and Policy Implications.* Toronto: Thompson Educational Publishing.

Jacobs, J. 1990. "Reassessing Mother Blame in Incest." *Signs: Journal of Women in Culture and Society* 15(3):500-14.

Jamieson, K. 1979. "Multiple Jeopardy: The Evolution of the Native Women's Movement." *Atlantis* 4(2):157-78.

Jenson, J. 1989. "Different but Not Exceptional: Canada's Permeable Fordism." *Canadian Review of Sociology and Anthropology* 26(1):69-94.

Jiwani, J. 1996. "B.C.'s lost opportunity to consider motherwork." *Vancouver Sun,* October 4, A23.

Johnson, A., S. McBride, and P. Smith, (eds.). 1994. *Continuities and Discontinuities: The Political Economy of Social Welfare and Labour Market Policy in Canada.* Toronto: University of Toronto Press.

Johnson, J. 1992. *Mothers of Incest Survivors: Another Side of the Story.* Bloomington: Indiana University Press.

Johnston, P. 1983. *Native Children and the Child Welfare System.* Toronto: Canadian Council on Social Development.

Kammerman, S. 1991. "Parental Leave and Infant Care: US and International Trends and Issues, 1978-1988." In J.S. Hyde and M.J. Essex (eds.), *Parental Leave and Child Care.* Philadelphia: Temple University Press.

Kammerman, S., and A. Kahn. Forthcoming. "Family Change and Family Policies in the US." In S. Kammerman and A. Kahn (eds.), *Family Change and Family Policies in Comparative Perspective.* Oxford: Oxford University Press.

_____. 1990. "Social Services for Children, Youth, and Families in the United States." *Children and Youth Services Review* 12(2):1-179.

Kangas, O., and J. Palme. 1992-93. "Statism Eroded? Labor-Market Benefits and Challenges to the Scandinavian Welfare States." *International Journal of Sociology* 22(4):3-24.

Keating, D.P., and J.F. Mustard. 1993. "Social Economic Factors and Human Development." In D. Ross et al. (eds.), *Family Security in Insecure Times: National Forum on Family Security.* Ottawa: Canadian Council on Social Development.

Kerstetter, S. 1997. "Fighting Child Poverty with Parental Work Income Supplements." In J. Pulkingham and G. Ternowetsky (eds.), *Child and Family Policies: Struggles, Strategies and Options.* Halifax: Fernwood.

Kesselman, J.R. 1994. "Public Policies to Combat Child Poverty: Goals and Options." In K.G. Banting and K. Battle (eds.), *A New Social Vision for Canada: Perspectives on the Federal Discussion Paper on Social Policy Reform.* Kingston: Queen's University, School of Policy Studies and Caledon Institute of Social Policy.

Kimelman, E. 1985. *No Quiet Place.* Final Report to the Honourable Muriel Smith Minister of Community Services. Winnipeg: Manitoba Community Services.

Kirsh, S. 1983. *Unemployment: Its Impact on Body and Soul.* Toronto: Canadian Mental Health Association.

_____.1992. "Mental Health and Unemployment." *Social Action Series.* Toronto: Canadian Mental Health Association.

Kitchen, B. 1992. "The Political Economy of Poor Mothers." *Canadian Woman Studies* 12(4):10-15.

_____. 1994. "Focus on the Child." In L. Bella, P. Rowe and D. Costello (eds.), *Rethinking Social Welfare: People, Policy, and Practice.* St. John's: Proceedings of the Sixth Biennial Social Welfare Policy Conference.

Kitchen, B., A. Mitchell, P. Clutterbuck, and M. Novick. 1991. *Unequal Futures: The Legacies of Child Poverty in Canada.* Toronto: Social Planning Council of Metropolitan Toronto.

Klein, B.W., and P.L. Rones. 1989. "A Profile of the Working Poor." *Monthly Labor Review* 112:3-13.

Kornberg, A., and H.D. Clarke. 1992. *Citizens and Community.* Cambridge: Cambridge University Press.

Krahn, H.J., and G.S. Lowe. 1993. *Work, Industry, and Canadian Society.* Scarborough: Nelson Canada.

Krane, J. 1990. "Explanations of Child Sexual Abuse: A Review and Critique from a Feminist Perspective." *Canadian Review of Social Policy* 25:11-19.

_____. 1994. "The Transformation of Women into Mother Protectors: An Examination of Child Protection Practices in Cases of Child Sexual Abuse." Unpublished doctoral dissertation. Toronto: University of Toronto.

_____. 1997. "Least Disruptive and Intrusive Course of Action . . . for Whom? Insights from Feminist Analysis of Practice in Cases of Child Sexual Abuse." In J. Pulkingham and G. Ternowetsky (eds.), *Child and Family Policies: Struggles, Strategies and Options.* Halifax: Fernwood.

Krane, J., and L. Davies. 1995. "Mother-Blame in Child Sexual Abuse: A Look at Dominant Culture, Writings, and Practices." *Textual Studies in Canada* 7:21-35.

Lajeunesse, T. 1993. *Community Holistic Circle Healing: Hollow Water First Nation.* Ottawa: Minister of Supply and Services.

Land, H. 1991. "Time to Care." In M. Maclean and D. Groves (eds.), *Women's Issues in Social Policy.* New York: Routledge.

Langille, D. 1988. "The Business Council on National Issues and the Canadian State." *Studies in Political Economy* 24:41-85.

Langille, D., and A. Ismi. 1996. "The Corporate Connection." *Canadian Perspectives* Autumn. Ottawa: Council of Canadians.

Lesemann, F., and R. Nicol. 1994. "Family Policy: International Comparisons." In Maureen Baker (ed.), *Canada's Changing Families: Challenges to Public Policy.* Ottawa: Vanier Institute of the Family.

Lewis, J. (ed.). 1993. *Women and Social Policies in Europe. Work, Family and the State.* Aldershot, England: Edward Elgar.

Lewis, R. 1996. "Warnings of an Explosion Point." *Maclean's* 109(46):4.

Leys, C., and M. Mendell. 1992. *Culture and Social Change.* Montreal: Black Rose Books.

Lindsay, C. 1992. *Lone-Parent Families in Canada: Target Groups Project.* Ottawa: Statistics Canada.

Little, B. 1996. "How the Earnings of the Poor Have Collapsed." *The Globe and Mail,*

February 12, A6.

Lochhead, C. 1997. "Identifying Low Wage Workers and Policy Options." In J. Pulkingham and G. Ternowetsky (eds.), *Child and Family Policies: Struggles, Strategies and Options.* Halifax: Fernwood.

Lochhead, C., and V. Shalla. 1996. "Delivering the Goods: Income Distribution and the Precarious Middle Class." *Perception* 20(Spring):15-20.

Lochhead, C., and R. Shillington. 1996. *A Statistical Profile of Urban Poverty.* Ottawa: Canadian Council on Social Development.

London-Edinburgh Weekend Return Group. 1979. *In and Against the State.* London: Pluto.

Loney, M. 1977. "A Political Economy of Citizen Participation." In L. Panitch (ed.), *The Canadian State: Political Economy and Political Power.* Toronto: University of Toronto Press.

Longclaws, L. 1994. "Social Work and the Medicine Wheel Framework." In B. Compton and B. Galaway (eds.), *Social Work Processes.* California: Brooks/Cole Publishing Company.

Low, W. 1996. "Wide of the Mark: Using 'Targeting' and Work Incentives to Direct Social Assistance to Single Parents." In. J. Pulkingham and G. Ternowetsky (eds.), *Remaking Canadian Social Policy: Social Security in the Late 1990s.* Halifax: Fernwood.

Loxley, J. 1981. "The Great Northern Plan." *Studies in Political Economy* 6:151-82.

Lubeck, S., and P. Garrett. 1991. "Child Care in America: Retrospect and Prospect." In E.A. Anderson and R.C. Hula (eds.), *The Reconstruction of Family Policy.* New York: Greenwood Press.

MacLeod, M., and E. Saraga. 1988. "Challenging the Orthodoxy: Towards a Feminist Theory and Practice." *Feminist Review* 28:16-55.

Macpherson, C.B. 1987. *The Rise and Fall of Economic Justice and Other Essays.* Oxford: Oxford University Press.

Mahon, R. 1977. "The Unequal Structure of Representation." In L. Panitch (ed.), *The Canadian State: Political Economy and Political Power.* Toronto: University of Toronto Press.

Mandell, N. 1988. "The Child Question: Links Between Women and Children in the Family." In N. Mandell and A. Duffy (eds.), *Reconstructing the Canadian Family: Feminist Perspectives.* Toronto: Butterworths.

Manitoba, Government of. 1982. *The Community Child Day Care Standards Act.* Chapter C-158. As amended.

_____. 1991. *Report of the Aboriginal Justice Inquiry of Manitoba.* Winnipeg: Queen's Printer.

_____. 1992. *The Desjarlais Inquest.* Winnipeg: Department of Justice.

_____. 1993. *The Child and Family Services Act.* 138/91. Amended December 1993.

Marlow, C. 1991. "Women, Children and Employment: Responses by the US and Great Britain." *International Social Work* 34:287-97.

Marsh, L.C. 1975. *Social Security for Canada.* Re-edited version of 1943 original. Toronto: University of Toronto Press.

Mayfield, M. 1990. "Parent Involvement in Early Childhood Programs." In I.M. Dovey (ed.), *Child Care and Education: Canadian Dimensions.* Toronto: Nelson Canada.

Maxwell, J. 1993. "Globalization and Family Security." In D. Ross et al. (eds.), *Family Security in Insecure Times: National Forum on Family Security.* Ottawa: Canadian

Council on Social Development.

McBride, S., and P. Shields. 1993. *Dismantling a Nation: Canada and the New World Order.* Halifax: Fernwood.

McCarthy, M. 1986. *Campaigning for the Poor: CPAG and the Politics of Welfare.* Beckenham: Croom Helm.

McDaniel, S.A. 1990. *Towards Family Policies in Canada with Women in Mind.* Feminist Perspectives, No. 17. Ottawa: Canadian Research Institute for the Advancement of Women.

_____. 1993. "Where the Contradictions Meet: Women and Family Security in Canada in the 1990s." In D. Ross et al. (eds.), *Family Security in Insecure Times. National Forum on Family Security.* Ottawa: Canadian Council on Social Development.

McFadden, E.J., and S.W. Downs. 1995. "Family Continuity: The New Paradigm in Permanence Planning." *Community Alternatives* 7(1):39-59.

McFate, K. 1991. "Poverty, Inequality and the Crisis of Social Policy. Summary of Findings." Unpublished paper prepared for the Joint Centre for Political and Economic Studies, Washington, DC.

McGilly, F. 1990. *Canada's Public Social Services.* Toronto: McClelland and Stewart.

McGrath, S. 1995. "The Role of Civil Society in the Process of Social Change: A Reconceptualization in the Context of Social Welfare." Comprehensive paper submitted in partial fulfillment of doctoral requirements in the Faculty of Social Work. Toronto, University of Toronto.

_____. 1997. "Child Poverty Advocacy and the Politics of Influence." In J. Pulkingham and G. Ternowetsky (eds.), *Child and Family Policies: Struggles, Strategies and Options.* Halifax: Fernwood.

McInnes, C. 1996. "BC Cutting Wrong Jobs, Analysts Feel." *The Globe and Mail,* November 12, A5.

McKenzie, B. 1994a. *Evaluation of the Pilot Project on Block Funding for Child Maintenance.* Winnipeg: West Region Child and Family Services.

_____. 1994b. "Decentralized Social Service: A Critique of Models of Service Delivery." In A. Johnson, S. McBride and P.J. Smith (eds.), *Continuities and Discontinuities: The Political Economy of Social Welfare and Labour Market Policy in Canada.* Toronto: University of Toronto Press.

_____. 1995. *Aboriginal Foster Care in Canada: A Policy Review.* Unpublished report for the Royal Commission on Aboriginal Peoples. Ottawa: Ontario.

_____. 1997. "Connecting Policy and Practice in First Nations Child and Family Services: A Manitoba Case Study." In J. Pulkingham and G. Ternowetsky (eds.), *Child and Family Policies: Struggles, Strategies and Options.* Halifax: Fernwood.

McKenzie, B., and P. Hudson. 1985. "Native Children, Child Welfare and the Colonization of Native People." In K.L. Levitt and B. Wharf (eds.), *The Challenge of Child Welfare.* Vancouver: University of British Columbia Press.

McKenzie, B., and V. Morrissette. 1993. "Aboriginal Child and Family Services in Manitoba: Implementation Issues and the Development of Culturally Appropriate Services." Unpublished paper presented at the Sixth Biennial Social Welfare Policy Conference, June 27-30. St. John's, Newfoundland.

McKenzie, B., E. Seidl, and N. Bone. 1995. "Child and Family Services Standards in First Nations: An Action Research Project." *Child Welfare* 74(3):633-53.

McQuaig, L. 1995. *Shooting the Hippo: Death by Deficit and Other Canadian Myths.* Toronto: Viking.

Melichercik, J. 1978. "Child Welfare in Ontario." In S. Yelaja (ed.), *Canadian Social Policy*. Waterloo: Wilfrid Laurier University Press.

Mendelson, M. 1995. "Not by Spending Cuts Alone." In Caledon In stitute of Social Policy, *Critical Commentaries on the Social Security Review*. Ottawa: Caledon Institute of Social Policy.

_____. 1996. "The Best Income Security System We Never Had." In D.P. Ross, et al. (eds.), *Family Security in Insecure Times, Perspectives (Volume II)*. Ottawa: Canadian Council on Social Development.

Mercredi, O. 1991. "Alternatives to Social Assistance in Indian Communities." In F. Cassidy and S.B. Seward (eds.), *Alternatives to Social Assistance in Indian Communities*. Toronto: Institute for Research on Public Policy.

Metcalf, D. 1981. *Low Pay, Occupational Mobility, and Minimum Wage Policy in Britain*. Washington, DC: American Enterprise Institute.

Metro Campaign 2000. 1995. *Child Poverty in Metropolitan Toronto: Report Card 1995*. Toronto: Metro Campaign 2000.

Miller, A. 1984. *For Your Own Good: Hidden Cruelty in Child-Rearing and the Roots of Violence*. Toronto: Collins Publishers.

Mimoto, H., and P. Cross. 1991. "The Growth of the Federal Debt." *Canadian Economic Observer* 3:1-17.

Minister of Supply and Services. 1985. *Report of the Royal Commission on the Economic Union and Development Prospects for Canada*. Volume 2. Ottawa: Minister of Supply and Services.

Ministerial Council on Social Policy Reform and Renewal. 1995. "Report to Premiers."

Mishra, R. 1984. *The Welfare State in Crisis: Social Thought and Social Change*. Great Britain: Wheatsheaf Books.

_____. 1990. *The Welfare State in Capitalist Society: Policies of Retrenchment and Maintenance in Europe, North America and Australia*. Toronto: University of Toronto Press.

Moroney, R.M. 1981. "Policy Analysis Within a Value Theoretical Framework." In R. Haskins and J. Gallagher (eds.), *Models for Analysis of Social Policy: An Introduction*. Norwood, NJ: Ablex.

Morris, A., and A. Wilczynski. 1994. "Mothers Who Kill Their Children." In H. Birch (ed.), *Moving Targets: Women, Murder and Representation*. Berkeley: University of California Press.

Morrissette, V. 1991. "Aboriginal Identity and Culturally Appropriate Services." Unpublished paper presented to University of Manitoba, Faculty of Social Work. Winnipeg.

Morrissette, V., B. McKenzie, and L. Morrissette. 1993. "Towards an Aboriginal Model of Social Work." *Canadian Social Work Review* 10(1):91-108.

Moscovitch, A. 1990. "Slowing the Steamroller: The Federal Conservatives, the Social Sector and Child Benefits Reform." In K.A. Graham (ed.), *How Ottawa Spends 1990-91: Tracking the Second Agenda*. Ottawa: Carleton University Press.

_____. 1996. "Canada Health and Social Transfer: What Was Lost?" *Canadian Review of Social Policy* 37:66-74.

Mullaly, R. 1993. *Structural Social Work: Ideology, Theory and Practice*. Toronto: McClelland and Stewart.

Myer, M.H. 1985. "A New Look at Mothers of Incest Victims." *Journal of Social Work and Human Sexuality* 3(2/3):47-58.

National Council of Welfare (NCW). 1992. *The 1992 Budget and Child Benefits.* Ottawa: Minister of Supply and Services.

_____ . 1993. *Incentives and Disincentives to Work.* Ottawa: Minister of Supply and Services.

_____ . 1994a. *A Blueprint for Social Security Reform.* Ottawa: Minister of Supply and Services.

_____ . 1994b. *Poverty Profile 1992.* Ottawa: Minister of Supply and Services.

_____ . 1995a. *Poverty Profile 1993.* Ottawa: Minister of Supply and Services.

_____ . 1995b. *The 1995 Budget and Block Funding.* Ottawa: Minister of Supply and Services.

_____ . 1996. *Poverty Profile 1994.* Ottawa: Minister of Supply and Services.

National Forum on Family Security. 1993. *Keynote Paper.* Ottawa: Canadian Council on Social Development.

Naylor, N. 1995. "Assessing the Possibility of a National Child Benefit Program." In M.D. Dooley, R. Finnie, S.A. Phipps and N. Naylor (eds.), *Family Matters: New Policies for Divorce, Lone Mothers, and Child Poverty.* Toronto: CD Howe Institute.

Nelson, K., and M. Landsman. 1992. *Alternative Models of Family Preservation: Family-Based Services in Context.* Illinois: Charles C. Thomas Publisher.

New, C., and M. David. 1985. *For the Children's Sake: Making Childcare More Than Women's Business.* London: Penguin.

Newman, N. 1996. "How Welfare Helps 'the Rest of Us.'" *Solutions* 1(1):1-2 (electronic newsletter available from *solutions@garnet.berkeley.edu*).

Novick, M., and R. Shillington. 1996. *Crossroads for Canada: A Time to Invest in Children and Families.* Toronto: Campaign 2000.

Offe, C. 1981. "Some Contradictions of the Modern Welfare State." Paper presented at the *Organization Economy Society: Prospects for the 1980s.* Brisbane: University of Queensland. July.

_____ . 1985. "New Social Movements: Challenging the Boundaries of Institutional Politics." *Social Research* 52(4):817-68.

O'Higgins, M., G. Schmauss, and G. Stephenson. 1990. "Income Distribution and Redistribution: A Microdata Analysis for Seven Countries." In T.M. Smeeding, M. O'Higgins and L. Rainwater (eds.), *Poverty, Inequality and Income Distribution in Comparative Perspective. The Luxembourg Income Study.* Washington: Urban Institute Press.

Olijnyk, Z. 1991. "Judge's Ruling: Native Groups Denied Jurisdiction." *Winnipeg Free Press,* May 10, A1, A5.

O'Neill, J. 1994. *The Missing Child in Liberal Theory: Towards a Covenant Theory of Family, Community, Welfare, and the Civic State.* Toronto: University of Toronto Press.

Ontario. 1984. *Bill 77: An Act Respecting the Protection and Well-Being of Children and Their Families.* Toronto: Queen's Printer.

Ontario Ministry of Community and Social Services. 1979. *A Discussion Paper. Child Welfare in Ontario: Past, Present and Future: A Study of Structure and Relationships.* Toronto: Ontario Ministry of Community and Social Services, Children's Services Division.

Orloff, A.S. 1993. "Gender and the Social Rights of Citizenship: The Comparative Analysis of Gender Relations and Welfare States." *American Sociological Review* 58(3):303-28.

Park, P., M. Brydon-Miller, B. Hall, and T. Jackson (eds.). 1993. *Voices of Change, Participatory Research in the United States and Canada.* Toronto: Ontario Institute for Studies in Education.

Parker, J. 1996. "Native Leaders Want Endorsement of Commission Recommendations." *The Star Phoenix,* November 22, B1.

Parton, C., and N. Parton. 1988/89. "Women, the Family and Child Protection." *Critical Social Policy* 24:38-49.

Pascall, G. 1986. *Social Policy: A Feminist Analysis.* New York: Tavistock.

Pashe, D. 1995. "Debit Audit Seen As Ploy." *Winnipeg Free Press,* February 9, A7.

Pateman, C. 1989. "The Public/Private Dichotomy." In C. Pateman (ed.), *Disorder of Women.* Stanford: Stanford University Press.

Pawley, H. 1996. "Devolution Favoured by BCNI Would Wreck Canada." Canadian Centre for Policy Alternatives, *Monitor* 3(5):1, 8.

Pearson, L. 1996. *Children and the Hill.* Fall. Ottawa: The Senate.

Pellegrin, A., and W. Wagner. 1990. "Child Sexual Abuse: Factors Affecting Victims' Removal from Home." *Child Abuse and Neglect* 14(1):53-60.

Perry, A. 1991. *Highgate Rise.* New York: Fawcett Crest.

Peters, S. 1995. *Exploring Canadian Values.* Ottawa: Canadian Policy Research Networks.

PG Anti-Poverty Coalition. 1996. *Prince George Poverty/Welfare Fact Sheet.* Prince George: UNBC, Child Welfare Research Centre.

Phipps, S.A. 1993. "International Perspectives on Income Support for Families with Children." Paper presented at Canadian Employment Research Forum Workshop on Income Support. September. Ottawa, Ontario.

_____. 1995a. "Canadian Child Benefits: Behavioural Consequences and Income Adequacy." *Canadian Public Policy* 21(1):20-30.

_____. 1995b. "Taking Care of Our Children: Tax and Transfer Options for Canada." In M.D. Dooley, R. Finnie, S.A. Phipps and N. Naylor (eds.), *Family Matters: New Policies for Divorce, Lone Mothers, and Child Poverty.* Toronto: CD Howe Institute.

_____. 1996. "Lessons from Europe: Policy Options to Enhance the Economic Security of Canadian Families." In D.P. Ross et al. (eds.), *Family Security in Insecure Times, Perspectives (Volume II).* Ottawa: Canadian Council on Social Development.

Phipps, S.A., and P.S. Burton. 1994a. *Sharing Within Families: Implications for the Distribution of Individual Well-Being in Canada.* Working Paper No. 94-07. Halifax: Dalhousie University, Department of Economics.

_____. 1994b. *What's Mine is Yours? The Influence of Male and Female Incomes on Patterns of Household Expenditure.* Halifax: Dalhousie University, Department of Economics.

Picot, G., and J. Myles. 1995. *Social Transfers, Changing Family Structure, and Low Income Among Children.* Product no. 11F0019E, no. 82. Ottawa: Statistics Canada, Analytical Studies Branch.

_____. 1996. "Children in Low-Income Families." *Canadian Social Trends* 42:15-19.

Pimento, B. 1985. *Native Families in Jeopardy: The Child Welfare System in Canada.* Occasional Papers in Social Policy Analysis (No.11). Toronto: University of Toronto, Department of Sociology and Education.

Popham, R., D.I. Hay and C. Hughes. Forthcoming. "Campaign 2000 to End Child Poverty: Building and Sustaining a Movement." In B. Wharf and M. Clague (eds.), *Community Organizing: Canadian Experiences.* Don Mills: Oxford University Press.

Premiers' Conference. 1996. "Social Policy Reform and Renewal." The 17th Annual Premiers' Conference. August 21-23. Jasper, Alberta.

Prentice, S. 1988. "Kids Are Not for Profit: The Politics of Childcare." In F. Cunningham et al. (eds.), *Social Movements/Social Change: The Politics and Practice of Organizing*. Toronto: Between the Lines.

_____. 1989. "Workers, Mothers, Reds: Toronto's Postwar Daycare Fight." *Studies in Political Economy* 30:115-41.

_____. 1993. "Militant Mothers in Domestic Times: Toronto's Postwar Childcare Struggle." Unpublished doctoral dissertation. Toronto: York University.

Prentice, S., and E. Ferguson. 1997. "'My Kids Come First': The Contradictions of Mothers' 'Involvement' in Childcare Delivery." In J. Pulkingham and G. Ternowetsky (eds.), *Child and Family Policies: Struggles, Strategies and Options*. Halifax: Fernwood.

Province of British Columbia. 1995. *BC Benefits: Renewing Our Social Safety Net*. Victoria: Queen's Printer.

_____. 1996a. *BC Benefits: The Initiative*. Victoria: Ministry of Social Services.

_____. 1996b. "Government Replaces Welfare for Youth with Job Search Assistance." *News Release*. Victoria. Premier's Office.

_____. 1996c. Ministry of Social Services. *Income Support Programs: Income Assistance Rates*. #PUB031. Victoria: Queen's Printer.

Pulkingham, J. 1995. "Investigating the Financial Circumstances of Separated and Divorced Parents: Implications for Family Law Reform." *Canadian Public Policy* 21(1):1-19.

_____. 1996. "Remaking the Social Divisions of Welfare: Gender, 'Dependency,' and UI Reform." Unpublished paper.

Pulkingham J., and G. Ternowetsky. 1996a. "The Changing Landscape of Social Policy and the Canadian Welfare State." In J. Pulkingham and G. Ternowetsky (eds.), *Remaking Canadian Social Policy: Social Security in the Late 1990s*. Halifax. Fernwood.

_____. 1996b. "Social Policy Choices and the Agenda for Change." In J. Pulkingham and G. Ternowetsky (eds.), *Remaking Canadian Social Policy: Social Security in the Late 1990s*. Halifax: Fernwood.

_____. 1997. *Child and Family Policies: Struggles, Strategies and Options*. Halifax: Fernwood.

Putnam, R.D. 1993. *Making Democracy Work*. Princeton: Princeton University Press.

Radbill, S. 1987. "Children in a World of Violence: A History of Child Abuse." In R. Helfer and R. Kempe (eds.), *The Battered Child*. Fourth edition. Chicago: The University of Chicago Press.

Red Horse, J. 1980. "American Indian Elders: Unifiers of Indian Families." *Social Casework* 61:490-93.

Remus, C. 1996. "Unraveling the Ties that Bind: The Decentralization of National Social Programs." *Briarpatch* 25(9):9-11.

Rich, A. 1977. *Of Woman Born: Motherhood as Experience and Institution*. London: Virago Press.

Rider, D. 1992. "Native Kids Can't Be Protected." *Winnipeg Sun,* May 26, 5.

Ringen, S. 1986. *Difference and Similarity: Two Studies in Comparative Income Distribution*. Stockhom: The Swedish Institute.

Rioux, M., and D.I. Hay, (eds.). 1993. *Well-Being: A Conceptual Framework*. Vancouver: Social Planning and Research Council (SPARC) of BC.

Rivers, B. 1993. "From Baby Snatcher to Family Builder: Paradigm Shifts in Child Welfare." In L. Bella (ed.), *Rethinking Social Welfare: People, Policy and Practice*. Proceedings of Sixth Biennial Social Welfare Policy Conference. June 27-30. St. John's, Newfoundland.

_____. 1996. "Children Living in Poverty." Letter. *The Globe and Mail,* November 26, A22.

Roeher Institute. 1993. *Social Well-Being: A Paradigm for Reform*. North York: Roeher Institute.

Rosenberg, H. 1988. "Motherwork, Stress, and Depression: The Costs of Privatized Social Reproduction." In B. Fox (ed.), *Family Bonds and Gender Divisions: Readings in the Sociology of the Family*. Toronto: Canadian Scholars Press.

Ross, D. et al. 1993. *Family Security in Insecure Times: National Forum on Family Security*. Volume I. Ottawa: Canadian Council on Social Development.

_____. 1996. *Family Security in Insecure Times. Perspectives*. Volume II. *Building a Partnership of Responsibility*. Volume III. Ottawa: Canadian Council on Social Development.

Ross, D., K. Scott, and M. Kelly. 1996. *Child Poverty: What Are the Consequences?* Ottawa: Canadian Council on Social Development.

Ross, D., and R. Shillington. 1989. *The Canadian Fact Book on Poverty 1989*. Ottawa: Canadian Council on Social Development.

Ross, D., E. Shillington, and C. Lochhead. 1994. *The Canadian Factbook on Poverty 1994*. Ottawa: Canadian Council on Social Development.

Ross, D.P. 1983. *The Family and the Fiscal System: Framework and Data for Evaluating Policies Affecting Families*. Ottawa: Family Service Canada.

Ross, R. 1992. *Dancing with a Ghost*. Toronto: Octopus Publishing Group.

Russo, N.F. 1979. "Overview: Sex Roles, Fertility, and The Motherhood Mandate." *Psychology of Women Quarterly* 4:7-15.

Sarlo, C. 1992. *Poverty in Canada*. Second edition. Vancouver: Fraser Institute.

Sassoon, A. 1987. "Women's New Social Role: Contradictions of the Welfare State." In A. Sassoon (ed.), *Women and the State: The Shifting Boundaries of Public and Private*. London: Hutchinson.

Saul, J.R. 1995. *The Unconscious Civilization*. Concord: Anansi.

Schaan, G. 1994. "Holistic Social and Health Services in Indian Communities." In A. Johnson et al. (eds.), *Continuities and Discontinuities. The Political Economy of Social Welfare and Labour Market Policy in Canada*. Toronto: University of Toronto Press.

Schmidt, G. 1997. "The Gove Report and First Nations Child Welfare." In J. Pulkingham and G. Ternowetsky (eds.), *Child and Family Policies: Struggles, Strategies and Options*. Halifax: Fernwood.

Schulz, P. 1978. "Day Care in Canada: 1850-1962." In K. Ross (ed.), *Good Day Care*. Toronto: Women's Educational Press.

Scott, K. 1996a. "The Dilemma of Liberal Citizenship: Women and Social Assistance Reform in the 1990s." *Studies in Political Economy* 50(Summer):7-36.

_____. 1996b. *The Progress of Canada's Children*. Ottawa: Canadian Council on Social Development.

Seligman, A.B. 1992. *The Idea of Civil Society*. New York: The Free Press.

Sgroi, S., L. Blick, and F. Porter. 1985. "A Conceptual Framework for Child Sexual Abuse." In S. Sgroi (ed.), *Handbook of Clinical Intervention in Child Sexual Abuse*. Toronto: Lexington Books.

Shapiro, S. 1977. "Parent Involvement in Daycare: Its Impact on Staff and Classroom Environment." *Child Welfare* 56(1):749-60.

Sharpe, A. 1996. "A Study of Contrasts: Income Distribution Trends in Canada and the United States." *CSLS News* 1:1-2. Ottawa: Centre for the Study of Living Standards.

Shillington, R. 1996. "The Tax System and Social Policy Reform." In J. Pulkingham and G. Ternowetsky (eds.), *Remaking Canadian Social Policy: Social Security in the Late 1990s*. Halifax: Fernwood.

Shimoni, R. 1992. "Parent Involvement in Early Childhood Education and Day Care." *Sociological Studies of Child Development* 5:73-95.

Sinclair, M. 1989. *Public Inquiry into the Administration of Justice and Aboriginal People*. Vancouver: The Western Workshop.

Smeeding, T., and L. Rainwater. 1991. "Cross-National Trends in Income Poverty and Dependency." Unpublished paper prepared for the Joint Center for Political and Economic Studies Conference on Poverty, Inequality, and the Crisis of Social Policy. Washington, DC: September 19–21.

Smith, B., and T. Smith. 1990. "For Love and Money: Women as Foster Mothers." *Affilia* 5(1):66-80.

Smith, R., and B. Vavrichek. 1992. "The Wage Mobility of Minimum Wage Workers." *Industrial and Labour Relations Review* 46(1):82-88.

Social Planning and Research Council of BC. 1992. *The Child Benefit: The 30 Cent Solution*. Brief submitted to the House of Commons Legislative Committee for Bill C-80. Vancouver: Social Planning and Research Council of BC.

_____. 1996. *Election '96 Fact Sheets: Jobs, Taxes, Health Care, Income, Aboriginal Treaties, Women*. Vancouver: Social Planning and Research Council of BC.

Social Planning Council of Metropolitan Toronto. 1985. "Economic Decline in Canada." In D. Drache and D. Cameron (eds.), *The Other Macdonald Report: The Consensus on Canada's Future that the Macdonald Commission Left Out*. Toronto: James Lorimer.

Spalter-Roth, R.M., and H.I. Hartmann. 1991. "Science and Politics and the 'Dual Vision' of Feminist Policy Research: The Example of Family and Medical Leave." In J.S. Hyde and M.J. Essex (eds.), *Parental Leave and Child Care*. Philadelphia: Temple University Press.

Stanford, J. 1996. "Discipline, Insecurity and Productivity: The Economics Behind Labour Market Flexibility." In J. Pulkingham and G. Ternowetsky (eds.), *Remaking Canadian Social Policy: Social Security in the Late 1990s*. Halifax: Fernwood.

Statistics Canada. 1992. *Labour Market Activity Survey 1988-1989-1990*. Longitudinal micro-data file, Catalogue MDF-3853b.

_____. 1996a. *Canadian Families: Diversity and Change* . Catalogue 12F0061XPE.

_____. 1996b. *Characteristics of Dual-earner Families, 1994*. Catalogue 13-215-XPB.

Strong-Boag, V. 1982. "Intruders in the Nursery: Childcare Professionals Reshape the Years One to Five, 1920-1940." In J. Parr (ed.), *Childhood and Family in Canadian History*. Toronto: McClelland and Stewart.

Struthers, J. 1994. *The Limits of Affluence*. Toronto: University of Toronto Press.

Swanson, J. 1994. "How the Government is Using Child Poverty to Mask Wider Poverty Issues." Action Canada Network. *Action Dossier* 40: 8-9.

Swanson, Jean. 1996. "The Poverty of Progress." In F.J. Tester, C. McNiven and R. Case (eds.), *Critical Choices, Turbulent Times: A Companion Reader on Canadian Social Policy Reform*. Vancouver: University of British Columbia, School of Social Work.

Swanson, Judy. 1996. "1 in 5 Children Lives in Poverty." *The Province,* November 19,

A4.

Swift, K. 1991. "Contradictions in Child Welfare: Neglect and Responsibility." In C. Baines, P. Evans and S. Neysmith (eds.), *Women's Caring: Feminist Perspectives on Social Welfare*. Toronto: McClelland and Stewart.

_____.1995. *Manufacturing "Bad Mothers": A Critical Perspective on Child Neglect*. Toronto: University of Toronto Press.

Taylor-Henley, S., and E. Hill. 1990. *Treatment and Healing, An Evaluation: Community Holistic Circle Healing*. Unpublished report.

Taylor-Henley, S., and P. Hudson. 1992. "Aboriginal Self-Government and Social Services: First Nations–Provincial Relationships." *Canadian Public Policy* 18(1):13-26.

Teichroeb, R. 1992. "Child Protection the Big Issue, McCrae Asserts." *Winnipeg Free Press* January 6, A1.

Ternowetsky, G. 1996. "Poverty Lines and Welfare Benefits in Prince George." *The Community Quilt* 1(2):3-4. Prince George: Community Social Planning Council.

Ternowetsky, G., and G. Riches. 1990. "Economic Polarization and the Restructuring of Labour Markets in Canada: The Way of the Future." In G. Riches and G. Ternowetsky (eds.), *Unemployment and Welfare: Social Policy and the Work of Social Work*. Toronto: Garamond.

Ternowetsky, G., and J. Thorn. 1991. *The Decline in Middle Incomes: Unemployment, Underemployment and Falling Living Standards in Saskatchewan*. Regina: University of Regina, Social Administration Research Unit.

Tester, K. 1992. *Civil Society*. London: Routledge.

Thomlison, R. 1984. *Case Management Review*. A Report Submitted to the Alberta Department of Social Services and Community Health. Calgary: University of Calgary.

Thorsell, W. 1996. "To Help Children in Poverty, Go to the Root of the Problem." *The Globe and Mail*, November 30, D8.

Time. 1994. "The Mother Who Killed Her Kids." *Time Magazine* 144(20):42.

Timpson, J. 1995. "Four Decades of Literature on Native Canadian Child Welfare: Changing Themes." *Child Welfare* 54(3):525-46.

Timpson, J. et al. 1988. "Depression in a Native Canadian Community in Northwestern Ontario: Sadness, Grief or Spiritual Illness?" *Canada's Mental Health* 36(2/3):5-8.

Tizya, R. 1992. "Aboriginal Governments and Power Sharing in Canada." In D. Brown (ed.), *Summary of Proceedings at the Institute of Intergovernmental Relations*. Toronto: Institute of Intergovernmental Relations.

Toupin, L. 1994. "New Directions in Social Policy: The Real People Behind the Statistics." In L. Bella, P. Rowe, and D. Costello (eds.), *Rethinking Social Welfare: People, Policy, and Practice*. St. John's: Proceedings of the Sixth Biennial Social Welfare Policy Conference.

Trocmé, N. 1991. "Child Welfare Services." In R. Barnhorst and L.C. Johnson (eds.), *The State of the Child in Ontario*. Toronto: Oxford University Press.

Trocmé, N., K. Tam, and D. McPhee. 1995. "Correlates of Substantiation of Maltreatment in Child Welfare Investigations." In J. Hudson and B. Galaway (eds.), *Child Welfare in Canada: Research and Policy Implications*. Toronto: Thompson Educational Publishing.

United Nations Development Program. 1990. *Human Development Report 1990*. New York-London: Oxford.

_____. 1991. *Human Development Report 1991*. New York-London: Oxford.

_____. 1992. *Human Development Report 1992*. New York-London: Oxford.

_____. 1993. *Human Development Report 1993*. New York-London: Oxford.

_____. 1994. *Human Development Report 1994*. New York-London: Oxford.

_____. 1995. *Human Development Report 1995*. New York-London: Oxford.

United States Department of Labor, Bureau of Labor Statistics. 1993. *Monthly Labor Review*. Table 25. April. Washington, DC: US Government Printing Office.

Ursel, J. 1992. *Private Lives, Public Policy: 100 Years of State Intervention in the Family*. Toronto: Women's Press.

Väisänen, I. 1992. "Conflict and Consensus in Social Policy Development: A Comparative Study of Social Insurance in Eighteen OECD Countries 1930-1985." *European Journal of Political Research* August (22):307-27.

Valpy, M. 1993. "The Myth of the Myth of Canadian Compassion." In D. Ross et al. (eds.), *Family Security in Insecure Times. National Forum on Family Security (Volume I)*. Ottawa: Canadian Council on Social Development.

Valpy, M. 1997. "A Down Payment, But Where Does it Lead." *The Globe and Mail*, February 20:A21.

Vancouver Sun. 1994: "Fix the System that Killed Matthew." *The Vancouver Sun*, May 3, A14.

_____. 1996a. "Child Poverty: Is the Solution More Taxes?" *The Vancouver Sun*, November 19, A15.

_____. 1996b. "Work, Not Taxes: Children Won't Emerge From Poverty Until Their Parents Have Decent Jobs." Editorial. *The Vancouver Sun*, November 20, A14.

Van Dijk, T. 1988. *News as Discourse*. Hillsdale, N.J.: Lawrence Eribaum Associates.

_____. 1993. "Principles of Critical Discourse Analysis." *Discourse and Society* 4(2):249-83.

Varga, D. 1991. "The Cultural Organization of the Childcare Curriculum: The University of Toronto's Institute of Child Study and Day Nurseries, 1890-1960." Unpublished doctoral dissertation. Toronto, University of Toronto, OISE.

Vickers, J., P. Rankin, and C. Appelle. 1993. *Politics As If Women Mattered*. Toronto: University of Toronto Press.

Vosko, L. 1996. "Irregular Workers, New Involuntary Social Exiles: Women and U.I. Reform." In J. Pulkingham and G. Ternowetsky (eds.), *Remaking Canadian Social Policy: Social Security in the Late 1990s*. Halifax: Fernwood.

Wald, M. 1982. "State Intervention on Behalf of Endangered Children: A Proposed Legal Response." *Child Abuse and Neglect* 6:3-45.

Wastasecoot, J. 1995. Editorial. *The First Perspective*. April:23.

Wattenberg, E. 1985. "In a Different Light: A Feminist Perspective on the Role of Mother in Father-Daughter Incest." *Child Welfare* 64(3):205-11.

Weller, M. 1996. Personal communication. Staff person, Fraser Institute.

Wennemo, I. 1994. *Sharing the Cost of Children*. Stockholm: Swedish Institute for Social Research.

West, E.G., and M. McKee. 1980. *Minimum Wages: New Issues in Theory, Evidence, Policy and Politics*. Ottawa: Minister of Supply and Services.

Westergard-Nielsen, N. 1994. "Wage Mobility in Denmark 1980-1990." Paper presented at the OECD conference on Employment Growth in the Knowledge Based Economy in Copenhagen. November 7-8.

Wharf, B. (ed.). 1979. *Community Work in Canada*. Toronto: McClelland and Stewart.

_____. 1989. *Toward First Nation Control of Child Welfare: A Review of Emerging*

Developments in B.C. Victoria: University of Victoria.

_____. 1992. *Communities and Social Policy in Canada.* Toronto: McClelland and Stewart.

_____. 1993a. "Rethinking Child Welfare." In B. Wharf (ed.), *Rethinking Child Welfare in Canada.* Toronto: McClelland and Stewart.

_____. 1993b. "The Constituency/Community Context." In B. Wharf (ed.), *Rethinking Child Welfare in Canada.* Toronto: McClelland and Stewart.

_____. 1995. "Organizing and Delivering Child Welfare Services: The Contributions of Research." In J. Hudson and B. Galaway (eds.), *Child Welfare in Canada: Research and Policy Implications.* Toronto: Thompson Educational Publishing.

Wharf, B., and M. Callahan. 1984. "Connecting Policy and Practice." *Canadian Social Work Review*:30-52.

Wilczynski, A. 1991. "Images of Women Who Kill Their Infants: The Mad and the Bad." *Women and Criminal Justice* 2:71-88.

Wilensky, H., and C. Lebeaux. 1965. *Industrial Society and Social Welfare.* New York: Macmillan.

Williams, F. 1989. *Social Policy: A Critical Introduction: Issues of Race, Gender and Class.* Cambridge: Polity Press.

Wills, G. 1995. *A Marriage of Convenience.* Toronto: University of Toronto Press.

Wilson, E. 1977. *Women and the Welfare State.* London: Tavistock.

Wineman, S. 1984. *The Politics of Human Services.* Montreal: Black Rose Books.

Winnipeg Council of First Nations. 1994. *Position Paper on the Dismantling of the Department of Indian Affairs and Urban Self-Government.* Presented at the Assembly of Manitoba Chiefs Conference on Self-Government. June. Winnipeg, Manitoba.

Winter, K. 1992. *The Day They Took Away Our Children: Ritualistic Abuse, Social Work and the Press.* Norwich: Social Work Monographs.

Wood, E.M. 1990. "The Uses and Abuses of Civil Society." In R. Miliband, L. Panitch and J. Saville (eds.), *Socialist Register.* London: Merlin Press.

Woolley, F., A. Vermaeten, and J. Madill. 1996. "Ending Universality: The Case of Child Benefits." *Canadian Public Policy* 22(1):24-39.

Wroe, A. 1988. *Social Work, Child Abuse and the Press.* Norwich: Social Work Monographs.

Yalnizyan, A. 1995. "Budget 1995: Open Intentions, Hidden Costs." *Social Infopac* 13(4). Toronto: Social Planning Council of Metropolitan Toronto.

Yeung, H. 1996. "Child Poverty: Poor Parents are Hard Pressed to Meet the Nutritional Needs of Their Children." *Focus on Children and Youth* 1(2):5.

York, C. 1991. *The Labor Movement's Role in Parental Leave and Child Care.* In J.S. Hyde and M.J. Essex (eds.), *Parental Leave and Child Care.* Philadelphia: Temple University Press.

York, G. 1991. "Coalition Stresses Plight of Poor Children." *The Globe and Mail,* November 22, A3.

Ziedenberg, J. 1996. "The Counter Revolution." *Canadian Dimension* 30(2):6-8.

Zyblock, M. 1996a. *Child Poverty Trends in Canada: Exploring Depth and Incidence from a Total Money Income Perspective, 1975 to 1992.* Working Paper W-96-1E. Ottawa: Human Resources Development Canada, Applied Research Branch.

_____. 1996b. *Individual Earnings Inequality and Polarization: An Exploration into Population Sub-Group Trends in Canada, 1981 to 1993.* Draft Working Paper. Ottawa: Human Resources Development Canada, Applied Research Branch.